Improving the Quality of
of
Patient Care

Alan Gillies

Lancashire Business School, Preston, UK

With contributions from

Nicola Ellis

Research, Information Management Research Group, Lancashire Business School, UK

and

Jan Barnsley, Louise Lemieux-Charles *and* **G. Ross-Barker**

Hospital Management Research Unit, Department of Health Administration, University of Toronto

JOHN WILEY & SONS
Chichester • New York • Brisbane • Toronto • Singapore

Copyright © 1997 by John Wiley & Sons Ltd,
Baffins Lane, Chichester,
West Sussex PO19 1UD, England

National   01243 779777
International   (+44) 1243 779777
e-mail (for orders and customer service enquiries):
cs-books@wiley.co.uk
Visit our Home Page on http://www.wiley.co.uk
or http://www.wiley.com

Other Wiley Editorial Offices

John Wiley & Sons, Inc., 605 Third Avenue,
New York, NY 10158-0012, USA

Jacaranda Wiley Ltd, 33 Park Road, Milton,
Queensland 4064, Australia

John Wiley & Sons (Canada) Ltd, 22 Worcester Road,
Rexdale, Ontario M9W 1L1, Canada

John Wiley & Sons (Asia) Pte Ltd, 2 Clementi Loop #02-01,
Jin Xing Distripark, Singapore 129809

Library of Congress Cataloging-in-Publication Data

Gillies, Alan.
    Improving the quality of patient care / Alan Gillies ; with
contributions from Nicola Ellis ... [et al.].
        p.   cm.
    Includes bibliographical references and index.
    ISBN 0-471-96647-9 (paper ; alk. paper)
    1. Medical care—Evaluation.   2. Medical Care—Quality control.
3. Hospital care—Evaluation.   4. Hospital care—Quality control.
5. Outcome assessment (Medical care)   I. Title.
    [DNLM: 1. Quality Assurance, Health Care.   2. Outcome and Process
Assessment (Health Care).   3. Medical Audit.   W 84.1 G481i 1997]
RA399.A1G54   1997
362.1'1—dc20
DNLM/DLC
for Library of Congress   96–25143
                                                              CIP

British Library Cataloguing in Publication Data

A catalogue record for this book is available from the British Library

ISBN 0-471-96647-9

Typeset in 11/13pt Palatino from the author's disks by Keytec Typesetting Ltd
Printed and bound in Great Britain by Biddles Ltd, Guildford and King's Lynn
This book is printed on acid-free paper responsibly manufactured from sustainable forestation, for which at least two trees are planted for each one used for paper production.

Contents

Preface

This book is designed to help people improve patient care. It is also written to give an honest account of the many techniques that exist, apparently to assist in this laudable aim. It covers theory, but includes much practical experience drawn from different countries, including the UK, USA and Canada. The practical element is presented both in the form of case studies and in guidance for future practice.

The book is principally intended to be read by practitioners, but it should appeal to managers as well. The first five chapters outline the theoretical foundations:

To begin with, Chapter 1 deals with the disturbingly complex question of What is healthcare? within the context of healthcare. It combines classical quality theory with practical illustrations from healthcare. Next, Chapter 2 outlines the historical and current context of quality within healthcare. It demonstrates that, with regard to quality, the present situation is a direct consequence of the history and current national health policy. Chapter 3 then examines the problems associated with trying to measure quality. The chapter develops a measurement framework for primary healthcare and illustrates how the overall performance may be shown graphically. Following this, Chapter 4 considers the development of classical process improvement ideas, and describes the ideas developed by the three gurus Deming, Juran and Crosby. It outlines the ISO9000 standard for quality management systems and looks at other techniques, such as quality circles. Finally, Chapter 5 looks at clinical audit, the principal improvement mechanism employed within the UK National Health Service (NHS). It shows how it may be seen to be a development of the classical process improvement ideas described in Chapter 4. It also shows how its growth is inextricably linked to the growth of computers.

The next three chapters are experiential in nature drawing on practical experience from the UK and North America:

To start with, Chapter 6 describes a major study of clinical audit practice in the Oxford health region. The study shows that current audit practice falls far short of that envisaged in the foundation legislation, and that the improvement process itself needs improvement. Chapter 7 then describes experience with occurrence screening as a quality mechanism. The chapter relates how the technique is predominant in the USA, and summarizes the debate about the effectiveness of the technique there. This is followed by details of one of the few UK studies based upon this technique. Finally, Chapter 8 looks at the use of indicators in the care of pre- and postnatal women in 18 Ontario hospitals. It is contributed by authors from the University of Toronto where the use of performance indicators has been studied in some detail.

The final two chapters are by way of conclusion:

Chapter 9 provides a practical guide to improving the improvement process. The method described is the subject of constant development and the version here is a snapshot of the 1996 vintage. The author welcomes enquiries about subsequent development. A complete paper-based method is under trial at the time of writing, and a paper describing the work won the 1996 Peter Reichertz Memorial Prize at the Medical Informatics Europe Conference. Lastly, Chapter 10 presents conclusions to the whole volume, looking at the principal themes, analysing the barriers to improvement, and suggesting some ways to reduce resistance.

Many people have helped with this book. It has been greatly enriched by the contributors. Numerous practitioners have helped through the medium of informal discussions, mostly within the Oxford University Postgraduate Medical Education and Training Department. The publishers have been a joy to work with, and Helen Tague has provided excellent clerical support at the University. I should also like to thank my wife, Jenny, for supplying patient experiences and asking awkward questions like What is quality, anyway?

In spite of all these contributions, the blame for any errors and omissions lies solely with me. Please send any comments to:

Alan Gillies
Professor of Information Management
University of Central Lancashire
Preston, Lancashire PR1 2HE, UK

or by Email to: a.c.gillies@uclan.ac.uk

CHAPTER 1

Defining the Quality of Healthcare

1.1 CHAPTER SUMMARY

The purpose of this book is to explore methods of improving patient care. In order to introduce real improvement it is necessary to establish current levels of performance, monitor the effect of change and then establish whether performance has improved.

This first chapter will establish the basis of our framework for assessing current performance. We shall explore the nature of patient care in terms of defining its quality. The chapter starts with the general problem of defining quality. It moves to consider the specific area of healthcare and its particular characteristics.

The concept of 'views' of quality is introduced through the specific example of the care of expectant mothers, considering the principal stakeholders and their views.

The general model of Garvin is then considered and its appropriateness for healthcare reviewed. This is followed by a model derived from Garvin's original, but tailored for healthcare. The chapter concludes with a consideration of the conflicts and constraints upon quality using this latter model as a basis.

1.2 A SIMPLE QUESTION WITH A DIFFICULT ANSWER

Some of the simplest questions are the most difficult to answer. 'What is quality?' ranks with the most difficult of them. In domains such as engineering, quality may be linked to tangible physical properties. However, in many other areas, and patient care in medicine is one of them, quality is intangible. As Kitchenham (1989) said in a different context, quality in such cases is 'hard to define, impossible to measure, easy to recognise'.

Quality is most easily recognized in its absence, and many public perceptions of healthcare are based upon measuring the absence of quality. Waiting times, waiting list sizes, even illness itself are all measurements of the absence of quality.

Traditionally, quality has been seen as 'the degree of excellence' (*Oxford English Dictionary*, 1990). This is an attractive definition but is insufficient for our purposes. The nature of 'excellence' must be considered in more detail to make the definition more effective. However, there is a more serious problem with this definition. Within a public health service context, it is necessary to consider the constraints upon excellence. Obviously, the primary constraint is budget, but others may exist, such as a shortage of specialist skills in clinical specialities or nursing.

An alternative definition of quality is provided by the International Standards Organisation (ISO, 1986):

> The totality of features and characteristics of a product or service that bear on its ability to satisfy specified or implied needs.

The standard definition associates quality with the ability of the product or service to fulfil its function. It recognizes that this is achieved through the features and characteristics of the product. Quality is associated both with having the required range of attributes and with achieving satisfactory performance within each attribute.

It is important to recognize some of the primary characteristics of quality:

(a) Quality is not absolute. It means different things in different situations. In the case of cars, a Mini and Rolls-Royce both represent quality in different ways. Quality cannot be measured upon a quantifiable scale in the same way as physical properties such as temperature or length.
(b) Quality is multidimensional. It has many contributing factors. It is not easily summarized in a simple, quantitative way.

Some aspects of quality can be measured objectively, such as time spent waiting to see a doctor; some may not, such as the quality of the doctor's manner during a consultation. The most easily measured criteria are not necessarily the most important. People are irrational beings, and the acceptability of their treatment may depend upon criteria which are very hard to define.

(c) Quality is subject to constraints. Assessment of quality in most cases cannot be separated from cost. However, cost may be wider than simple financial cost: it refers to any critical resources such as people, tools and time. Some resources will be more constrained than others, and where there is a high demand for a resource that is heavily constrained, the availability of that resource will become critical to overall quality.

(d) Quality is about acceptable compromises. Where quality is constrained and compromises are required, some quality criteria may be sacrificed more acceptably than others; e.g. comfort may be sacrificed before productivity. Those criteria that can least afford to be sacrificed may be regarded as critical attributes. They are often a small subset of the overall set of quality criteria.

(e) Quality criteria are not independent. The quality criteria interact with each other causing conflicts. For example, the greater the number of patients assigned to a clinic, the longer the waiting time during the clinic, but the shorter the waiting time to get an appointment. In this case, a conflict exists between the two desirable attributes.

(f) Acceptable quality changes over time. Progress in clinical practice and improvements in care mean that levels of performance deemed to be satisfactory are constantly being raised. This is an increase in both actual capability and in public expectation.

1.3 DEFINITIONS FROM WITHIN MEDICINE

The problem of defining quality in medical terms is the complexity of the issue. Any domain where we are dealing with people rather than artefacts is infinitely more complex. This has caused many authors to say that looking at improving healthcare through a quality assurance model derived from manufacturing industry is inappropriate:

> Human well-being and the health care industry which deals with it are infinitely more complex than production lines. (Crombie et al, 1993)

As far as it goes, this statement is fine; but quality assurance is now applied in many different organizational and service contexts which face many of the same issues as healthcare. An example is education.

The difficulty is in not oversimplifying the issues. This is particularly true when we seek to express the quality of healthcare in terms of simple quantitative measures.

For example, one traditional measure of healthcare is morbidity data. Many such measures tend to emphasize issues of quantity rather than quality. This tends to make clinicians uncomfortable who tend to evaluate themselves in terms of the quality of patients' lives rather than the quantity of it.

In practice, most writers in the clinical domain choose not to define quality at all, unless dealing with a very specific and tightly defined domain. For example, the definition of clinical audit provided by the Department of Health states that it is:

> the systematic, critical analysis of the quality of medical care, including the procedures used for diagnosis and treatment, the use of resources and the resulting outcome and quality of life for the patient. (DoH, 1990)

This definition contains the phrases 'quality of medical care' and 'quality of life' but nowhere defines what is meant by these terms. There is a broad consensus about general characteristics associated with these terms; but at a detailed level, different clinicians and other interested parties, not least patients, are likely to disagree.

Therefore, rather than attempt a reductionist definition we shall consider different views of the quality of patient care in a specific context. The next section considers the situation of the care of mothers, from antenatal to postnatal.

1.4 VIEWS OF QUALITY

We shall start by recognizing that quality is a multidimensional construct. Therefore, it is perhaps inevitable that it has been classified according to a number of 'views' or perspectives. We shall represent this by a visual analogy (Fig. 1.1).

These views are often diverse and may conflict with each other. Each view comes from a particular context, and any single view tends to give us only a partial picture. The views identified tend to be stereotypical. For example, a distinction is commonly made within the health service context between the clinicians or professionals and the managers or administrators. The views are generally presented in adversarial pairs such as professionals versus administrators. Such comparisons are usually loaded by the terminology used.

Obviously, there are more than two people involved in any

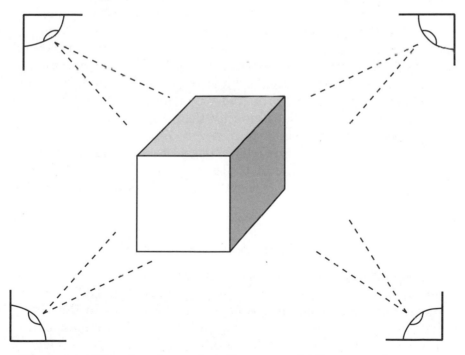

Figure 1.1 Visual analogy of quality as a multidimensional construct

healthcare procedure. The care of postnatal patients is particularly interesting for two reasons:

- it involves an unusually large number of people in different roles dealing with the patient
- the patient is generally not ill.

We shall consider each of the following roles and their view of quality:

- mother
- hospital midwife
- doctor
- community midwife

- baby
- unit manager
- mother's partner.

The Mother

The mother's view of the quality of her experience will depend upon two factors: a successful outcome and a positive experience before, during and after the birth. The duality of this view is emphasized by the fact that most mothers are not ill. Obviously at some points, these views are reinforcing. A simple and successful birth will encourage a positive view of the whole experience. However, some procedures which may be deemed clinically desirable to maximize the probability of a successful outcome may be highly invasive and disturbing for the mother.

Increasingly, the separation between these aspects is being questioned as it is recognized that clinical outcomes are influenced by a patient's general state of well-being. This increases the need to take account of what have been traditionally considered as non-clinical aspects of care.

The Hospital Midwife

The hospital midwife is in fact responsible for most births. The multidisciplinary approach which is being recognized in many clinical specialties as desirable has been the reality in delivering babies for a long time. The hospital midwife's prime responsibility is for a successful outcome for mother and baby. Their view of quality is complicated by their dual responsibility to both mother and baby. Increasingly, they are also being influenced by a need to demonstrate that all eventualities were considered in the light of possible litigation in the event of problems. This is a theme to which we shall return later.

The Doctor

Doctors are generally only involved significantly in births that have clinical complications. One doctor remarked that this made her an awful expectant mother as she had only ever witnessed difficult births. This, coupled with the fact that the doctor carries ultimate responsibility for any clinical problems, will tend to emphasize a view of quality based upon clinical outcomes.

The Community Midwife

The community midwife may be involved at the birth in the event of a home birth, but is more likely to be responsible for the daily postnatal care of mother and baby. The community midwife tends to avoid the worst clinical complications, and therefore can afford to pay more attention to patients' comfort. Generally involved postnatally, the midwife will also deal overtly with mother and baby.

The Baby

The baby, although unable to express a view, is the focus of at least half the care provided. Once again, there are clinical and experiential aspects of the quality of care received. However, the clinical aspects often dominate as the baby is not able to vocalize objections to treatments that may be thought clinically desirable, but are unpleasant for the baby.

The Unit Manager

The manager of the unit has the job of ensuring the quality of patient care delivered. Crucially, the manager has to weigh the needs of all patients rather than individuals. Decisions have to be taken in the light of available resources, and this means having to balance the quality of care against the quantity.

The Mother's Partner

The partner generally has a direct and indirect interest in the process, although the roles may be distinct. As the father of the child, he has a direct interest in the successful birth of the offspring. As the mother's partner he has an interest in the mother's health and happiness. Decisions to exclude partners from parts of the process, particularly at the antenatal stage, on the grounds of clinical expediency can lead to dissatisfaction and resentment.

1.5 MODELLING VIEWS OF QUALITY

Garvin's (1984) Model

Within the general management context, Garvin (1984) has suggested a model in terms of five different views of quality (Fig. 1.2). The meaning of Garvin's views are summarized in Table 1.1 on p.10. We shall now consider these views in more detail, within the context of healthcare.

Garvin's Transcendent View

This view relates quality to innate excellence. Another word for this might be 'elegance'. This is the classical definition of quality, in tune with the *Oxford English Dictionary*. It is impossible to quantify and is difficult to apply in a meaningful sense to healthcare. An attempt to build in a high degree of innate excellence to healthcare is likely to be constrained by resources. Seeking to build healthcare along these lines is inevitably expensive, and thus resource constraints will tend to emphasize the value-based view, described below, rather than the transcendent view.

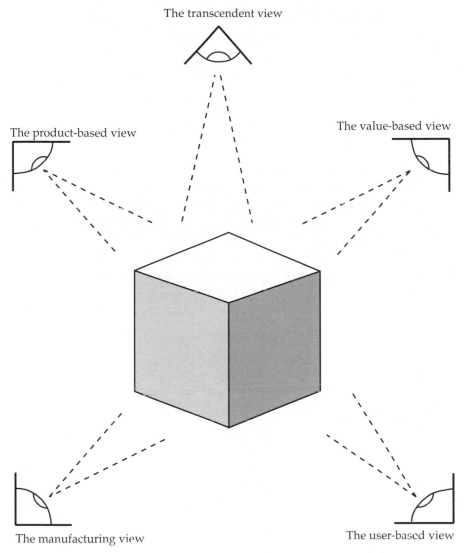

Figure 1.2 Garvin's model: five views of quality

Garvin's Product-Based View

This view is the economist's view: the higher the quality, the higher the cost. The basis for this view is that it costs money to provide a higher quality. This is a commonly held view about

Table 1.1 Summary of Garvin's views of quality

View	Meaning
Transcendent	Absolute excellence
Product-based	Higher quality means higher cost
User-based	Fitness for purpose
Manufacturing	Conformance to specification
Value-based	Quality at a specific price

healthcare. Better care and quicker access to services are commonly linked to more doctors, nurses and hospital beds. However, in certain areas, better practice may also be cheaper. Examples of this may be found in screening programmes where health screening (e.g. for blood pressure, cervical cancer and child immunization) can actually save money in the long term by keeping people healthy rather than treating people when they get ill.

Also, the growing practice of clinical audit is highlighting areas where practice can be improved without necessarily increasing costs.

This is the classic 'quality is free' argument proposed by the likes of Crosby (1986) but translated from manufacturing to healthcare. Crosby argues that by changing practice and reducing wastage, savings can be achieved in manufacturing which outweigh the costs of setting up the new procedures.

However, unfortunately, this is by no means universal. Many improved practices will involve new technology requiring investment. Once wastage is removed, improvements in waiting lists can only be achieved by more resources.

Many of the screening programmes which are cost effective in the long term are expensive in the short term. For example, the growth in screening programmes in the UK has driven up computerization rates amongst family doctors from around 25% to 90%. This represents a major investment whose cost must be set against the savings as illness is reduced.

Further, if screening programmes are justified on cost grounds alone, then programmes advantageous to health but less advantageous on cost grounds (e.g. breast cancer screening) may be marginalized. From a health perspective, it is still better to prevent illness rather than treat it, but this case conforms to Garvin's product-based view, i.e. higher quality of care costs more.

Garvin's User-Based View

This view, first championed by Juran in the 1940s, is traditionally expressed as fitness for purpose. It is sometimes represented as patient satisfaction. This can, however, be a simplification.

Fitness for purpose implies that the service provided meets the needs of patients. Thus, it certainly applies to aspects of performance such as waiting times, access to services and patient satisfaction. However, overall fitness for purpose is compromised if waiting times are reduced by emphasizing the treatment of conditions that are quick and easy to treat at the expense of more seriously ill patients.

It is also compromised if waiting times are reduced at the expense of reducing the effectiveness of treatment provided leading to an increase in readmissions. Many measures currently applied to the NHS which purport to measure NHS fitness for purpose (e.g. waiting times, waiting list sizes, number of patients treated) actually measure the quantity of healthcare provided rather than the quality.

Garvin's Manufacturing View

The manufacturer's view measures quality in terms of conformance to requirements. A simple example might be the dimensions of a component: the specification will state both the required dimensions and the tolerance that will be acceptable.

The manufacturing view emerges in healthcare in a number of ways. The first is the introduction of protocols and standards for specific clinical procedures. These may be regarded as specifications. In the UK, one of the stated outcomes of the clinical audit process is the introduction of standards to disseminate 'best practice'.

However, the setting of such standards is by no mean universal; a report on audit practice in the Oxfordshire Health Authority revealed that only 46% of audits were claimed to result in the setting of standards. Evaluation of 75 published audits indicated a 41% uptake. As published audits, these may be expected to show a higher uptake than the whole, suggesting that the real figure may be lower.

In practice, it is rarely possible to provide guidelines which embody 'best practice'. Guidelines will prevent bad practice and can lead to uniform improvements where existing practice is flawed. However, best practice generally requires skills and judgement which are not easily enshrined in deterministic procedures. Thus the result of guidelines can be problem avoidance rather than promotion of excellence.

Best practice requires the exercising of judgement, rather than following a deterministic procedure. The biggest threat to this lies in the increasing threat of malpractice suits. This encourages doctors to view quality in terms of meeting a specification. If the specification is met, the doctor has fulfilled his or her obligation, even if the patients' aspirations are not met.

Garvin's Value-Based View

In a business context, this is the ability to provide what the customer requires at a price that they can afford. In a public health service, the customer is ultimately the taxpaying public represented by the government. A value-based view of quality assesses the cost-effectiveness of a service or treatment.

The value-based view is the antithesis of the transcendent view, because it links quality to cost. Within the management of quality in the NHS context, this is often the crucial view. It is also what tends to give NHS management a bad name in the eyes of the public, as it recognizes that quality is ultimately resource-limited. Although there are cases where better healthcare costs less not more as described above, in general this is not the case.

An Alternative Model

Garvin's model is not necessarily appropriate for healthcare. For example, the manufacturing view which is dominant in many areas of traditional quality management is of limited use. The author therefore proposes an alternative view-based model of quality for healthcare (Fig. 1.3).

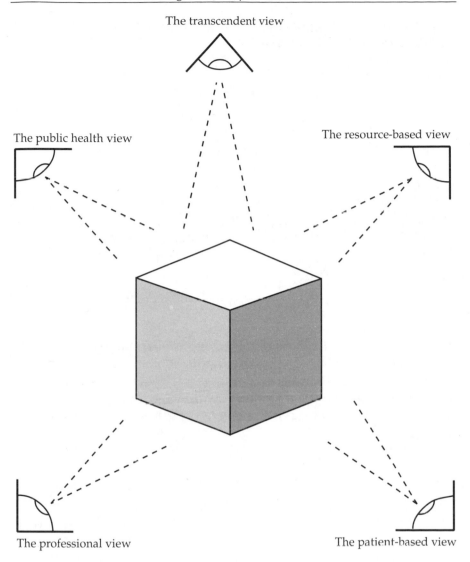

Figure 1.3 A view-based model of the quality of patient care

The Transcendent View

This view is the same as Garvin's. It is included because it is such a deeply ingrained view of quality. It is of little help in analysing the problem of improving the quality of patient care. However, it

is important to recognize its crucial place in many people's understanding of the nature of quality.

The Public Health View

This view is based upon the idea that the quality of patient care is
demonstrated by the health of the nation. It is the view at the heart
of the UK government's strategy document *Health of the Nation*
which sets targets for key areas of health to be achieved by the
end of the decade.

A key element of this view is that quality of care is reflected in
maintaining and restoring health rather than through treating
illness. This view may be seen as a strategic view of the quality of
patient care.

The Resource-Based View

The resource-based view says that the quality of patient care is the
maximum care that can be obtained for the resources allocated by
the country to public healthcare. Thus it is concerned with the
effectiveness of patient care, reduction of waste and promotion of
best practice measured in terms of value for money. This may be
thought of as the management view, at both an operational and a
strategic level.

The Professional View

This view emphasizes clinical outcomes and clinical expertise. It
sets a successful clinical outcome as the primary measure of
success. Traditionally, it has emphasized the central role of the
doctor. It is increasingly coming to promote a team-based approach. However, some doctors may use a narrow form of this
view to resist change in this direction. It is a view associated with
doctors and other clinical professionals.

The Patient-Based View

The patient-based view says that the patients' overall well-being
and satisfaction is crucial. It tends to an individualistic view rather

than a collective vision, as the needs of each patient may be different and conflict under the resource-based view with the needs of other patients. It may in certain cases conflict with the professional view as well. However, many professionals, placing their patients' needs as their prime objective, will subscribe to this view, although expressing it in a different way from the patients they seek to serve.

These views are necessarily stereotypical, as any model must represent a subset of reality. They are intended to be less stereotypical than a reductionist definition and more appropriate to healthcare than Garvin's general model. We shall return to them in later chapters.

1.6 CONFLICTS AND CONSTRAINTS

There is an extra degree of complexity inherent in our model which arises from the relationships which exist between each view of quality. It is suggested that each of the views except the transcendent view is in dynamic equilibrium with the others. The equilibrium is dynamic because many improvements as perceived from one point of view may degrade quality when perceived from another view. Each of the other four contributes to the transcendent view.

The dynamic equilibrium may be thought of in terms of a variety of conflicts between different views (Fig. 1.4).

The most commonly considered conflict is between cost and quality, or in terms of our views between the resource-based view and the public health view. Any improvements which can impact positively on more than one view without negatively impacting elsewhere are particularly attractive. Some of the screening programmes mentioned earlier are in this category.

However, there are other conflicts at work between the different views. There is a significant and growing conflict between patient and professional based views. A better informed public arising from a more patient-centred approach argues more strongly for their rights and attacks the traditionally unquestioned expertise of the professionals.

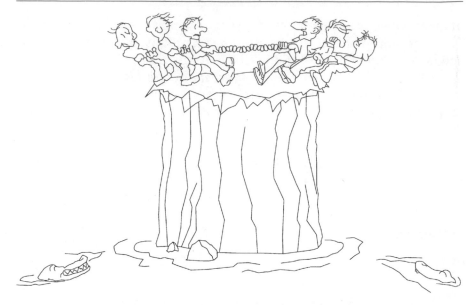

Figure 1.4   There may be conflicts between different views

Part of this is a growing awareness of the right of patients to make charges of negligence in cases where things go wrong. This has a number of consequences, but one is that doctors may take courses of action in order to protect them against malpractice suits rather than for patient-centred reasons. This will then tend to reduce the quality in terms of the patient-based approach. This has been seen more in the USA, where litigation is much more common than in the UK.

An example may be seen in the behaviour of American obstetricians, who in the face of increasing incidence of malpractice suits over birth canal deliveries opted for an increased number of caesarean section deliveries. In spite of the increased risk to patients, this was less likely to lead to a lawsuit. At its peak, this trend led to approximately 50% of births being delivered in this way. However, this was followed by a series of lawsuits which alleged unnecessary caesarean operations, which in turn reduced the number of operations. This slightly bizarre example illustrates the dynamic equilibrium which exists between different views of quality.

In an ideal world, all views would be satisfied, leading to the transcendent view of quality. However, in the real world, all of the others exist in different degrees of tension with each other. This is what makes a discussion of the quality of patient care so difficult and makes a multidimensional treatment essential.

1.7　REFERENCES

Crombie, I. K., Davies, H. T. O., Abraham, S. C. S. & du V. Florey, C. (1993) *The Audit Handbook: Improving Healthcare Through Clinical Audit.* Chichester: Wiley.

Crosby, P. B. (1986) *Quality is Free.* Maidenhead: McGraw-Hill.

Department of Health (1990) *Framework for Information Systems: Overview* (Working for Patients Working Paper 11). London: HMSO.

Garvin, D. (1984) What does quality mean? *Sloan Management Review*, **4**, 124–131.

International Standards Organisation (1986) *ISO 8042: Quality Vocabulary.* Geneva: ISO (available from BSI, London).

Kitchenham, B. (1989) Software quality assurance. *Microprocessors and Microcomputers*, **13**(6), 373–81.

CHAPTER 2

The Development of Quality Assurance Within Healthcare

2.1   CHAPTER SUMMARY

This chapter traces the development of quality assurance (QA) ideas from the 1850s to the current day. It considers the principal ideas and techniques, identifying three main approaches found in modern healthcare quality assurance.

The main approaches are characterized as top-down, bottom-up and process accreditation. The advantages and disadvantages of each are discussed.

The chapter then considers the provision of healthcare in a modern public health service, taking as an example the NHS with all the reforms that have been introduced over the last ten years.

Issues introduced here are developed in greater detail in later chapters.

2.2   THE ORIGINS OF QUALITY ASSURANCE IN HEALTHCARE

One of the most famous early examples of quality assurance activity in healthcare is the story of Florence Nightingale during the Crimean War. During the siege of Sebastopol in January 1855, British deaths occurring in the hospitals reached appalling levels, with 3168 in one month. Of these, 2761 were caused by infectious diseases whilst only 83 died from their wounds (Cohen, 1984).

Even then, healthcare was a contentious political issue. A vote of censure was passed on the government by 157 votes, bringing it down. As part of the response to the situation, Florence Nightingale was sent out to provide nursing care with a team of nurses.

The effect of changes introduced by Nightingale was remarkable. Within six months, the death rate had fallen from 40% of soldiers admitted to 2% (Crombie et al, 1993). Little of this was achieved by the traditional nursing immortalized in Nightingale's *Lady of the Lamp*: the improvements were due to practical improvements in sanitation arrangements:

- establishment of kitchens in her own premises
- establishment of an effective laundry service
- provision of adequate numbers of chamber pots.

Another factor which is recorded in this experience is the opposition of many of the doctors (Smith, 1950). Nightingale overcame some of this opposition by a mixture of careful documentation and a liberal use of her influence and contacts back home. However, she also recognized the need to sell the changes to the doctors as being in their own best interests.

A different approach is illustrated by a report for the Carnegie Foundation in 1910 by Flexner (Lembcke, 1967). This documented the poor standards of training provided by medical schools of the time. Flexner made a careful study of the problem and his detailed analysis led to some reforms. Medical training was moved to universities and given a proper theoretical foundation. The American College of Surgeons was formed in 1913 to accredit surgeons and improve standards.

Flexner's pioneering study was followed by a larger study of non-teaching hospitals in 1916 by Bowman (Roberts et al, 1987). The survey found that only 13% of large hospitals met minimum standards. This was considered shocking enough to prevent publication of the results.

However, it did lead to the establishment of minimum standards of care and to a list of accredited hospitals which met them. This was the start of a programme of hospital accreditation which was to lead to the later establishment of the Joint Commission on Accreditation of Hospitals.

A third strand of healthcare quality assurance may be seen in the national programmes in the UK and the US developed after the Second World War.

From 1952, data were collected on maternal mortality in England on a voluntary basis (Godber, 1976). The study was important because it focused on reasons for inadequate care rather than simply recording incidences. This study formed the basis of similar studies in other parts of the UK and Australasia. It may also be seen to provide many of the characteristics of modern investigations:

- it focuses on improvement rather than recording current practice
- guidelines were produced to improve care
- compliance was voluntary
- standard data collection forms were used
- the study was evolutionary and ongoing.

However, it was a voluntary initiative. In this it may be contrasted with the American Professional Standards Review Organizations (PSROs) established by legislation in 1972. The purpose of the programme was to monitor the hospital stay of every Medicare and Medicaid patient. Huge amounts of data were gathered at great expense. The programme faced many problems (Jonas & Rosenberg, 1986):

- speed of introduction
- scale
- cost
- quality of data, and verification thereof
- doctor opposition and consequent failure to change practice.

These three historical developments illustrate the three main strands of quality assurance activity in healthcare which we shall characterize as bottom-up, process accreditation and top-down. In the next section we shall explore the relative strengths and weaknesses of modern implementations of each approach.

2.3 APPROACHES TO QUALITY ASSURANCE IN THE CLINICAL CONTEXT

Top-down

In this approach, quality assurance is imposed from above. Procedures to assure quality within healthcare are defined by external legislation, usually at national, state or provincial level. Healthcare providers are required to provide data about the delivery of services. The system is made to work by sanctions against those who do not provide the required data. There are several potential advantages of this approach.

- *Consistency.* If QA procedures are imposed from above, then consistent procedures can be employed across different hospitals or regions. Results can then be compared for different hospitals and league tables compiled.
- *Strategic planning.* The availability of national performance figures allows for proper strategic planning to correct deficiencies in both healthcare procedures and provision.
- *Independent scrutiny.* Since the procedures are imposed from outside the immediate situation, they can be scutinized independently.

There are, however, major problems as illustrated by the PSRO programme described above.

- *Complexity and cost.* The complexity and size of healthcare delivery means that an effective and comprehensive QA procedure of this type is prohibitively expensive.
- *Practitioner resistance.* All imposed programmes will meet with some resistance. The power of the medical profession is such that it is unlikely to succeed in the face of such opposition (Fig. 2.1).
- *Data collection.* Data collection is crucial to the success of this type of programme. There are several problems. Data collection will depend upon practitioner cooperation, unlikely in the face of an imposed programme. Where data are collected, they may be of variable quality. Data verification may not be possible or practicable.

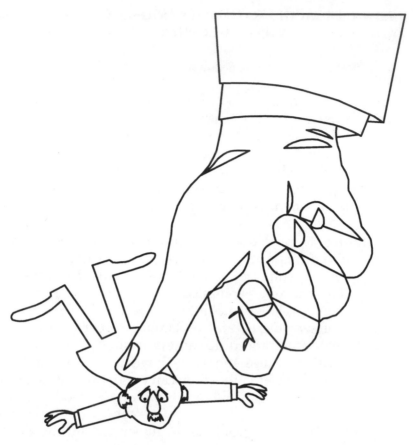

Figure 2.1   Top-down quality assurance can be viewed as an imposition

- *Failure to implement good practice.* It is a characteristic of such programmes that they tend to eliminate errors, but do not positively encourage good practice, since they actively discourage professionals from using professional judgements to depart from prescriptive procedures to improve the quality of care.
- *Focus upon ease of measurement.* It is a characteristic of such programmes that they emphasize the measurement of aspects of the quality of care. Measurement is often driven by what *can* be measured rather than what *should* be measured. Thus factors such as waiting times are often emphasized. The way that they are measured can further distort the measurement process.

Within the NHS Patient's Charter, for example, an external quality standard is imposed which requires patients to be seen within 30 minutes. The standard is often breached. However, patients would generally rather be seen after 35 minutes and given correct and helpful treatment, than be seen in under 30 minutes by perhaps an inexperienced or inappropriate person and given incorrect treatment.

Process Accreditation

In this approach, the processes by which healthcare is delivered and the associated QA procedures are documented. The documentation should cover:

- the scope of activities: what is done
- the procedures used: how it is done
- quality standards: how well it is done
- verification procedures: how you know how well it is done.

The documented procedures are then checked against external standards. If the documented procedures are appropriate, then the actual procedures will be checked by inspection by an external body.

This type of approach is typified by the ISO9000 standard for quality management systems, which is widely accepted as a quality mechanism in many business and manufacturing organizations. It is increasingly being adopted by service organizations, and is being sought by parts of the public healthcare system that find themselves in competition with commercial firms (e.g. for technical support and equipment servicing).

The process of scrutiny may be carried out by a first, second or third party:

- *First party.* This is self assessment and generally is only valuable as a precursor to external scrutiny.
- *Second party.* In this type of assessment, procedures are scrutinized by a specific customer. In a healthcare system such as the NHS, where the system is divided into purchasers and provi-

ders, then scrutiny of a provider would typically be carried out by a purchaser when purchasing healthcare services.

• *Third party*. In this type of assessment, an independent standards body is brought in to scrutinize procedures. Thus in the case of ISO9000 certification, a range of bodies are licensed to provide certification to show that the organization's quality management procedures meet the requirements of one of the ISO9000 series of standards.

Process accreditation, which is almost universal in other sectors, has specific applications in healthcare and has been historically significant through the various hospital accreditation programmes.

The approach has its own specific advantages. It offers an independent method of scrutiny, that uses a sampling technique to provide a cost-effective approach. Verification is based upon a snapshot of a sample of procedures, though future return visits are essential to ensure that quality is maintained.

There are disadvantages to the approach. First, it emphasizes consistency of approach over actual merit. Thus procedures must be defined and be able to handle 'non-conformances'. However, this does not necessarily require improvement in practice. Indeed, there can be a positive disincentive to improve since accredited organizations often feel that they have 'arrived' and do not need to improve further.

Secondly, if a generic quality management standard such as the ISO9000 series is used, then there is no direct assessment of the quality of the clinical procedures themselves, only the quality assurance and management procedures. Also, the inspection team are unlikely to be clinicians. The use of these standards is explored in more detail in Chapter 4.

Bottom-up

Bottom–up approaches start from the viewpoint that the best people to understand a process are the people who carry it out on a day by day basis. These may be doctors, nurses or managers.

Clinical audit as implemented in the NHS is an example of a 'bottom-up' technique. It is locally controlled and implemented.

The majority of studies are clinician-led. However, there are other techniques used particularly in business and manufacturing which are focused more on capturing 'front line' expertise in improving quality, such as quality circles. These are explored in Chapter 4. The advantages of bottom-up approaches are:

- *Local ownership.* If the practitioners feel that they are responsible for quality they are most likely to adopt changes which result from the quality assurance or improvement procedures.
- *Local expertise.* As stated above, the practitioners are likely to have expertise both about the job and about the defects in current procedures.
- *Effective targeting.* Arising from both the above considerations, resources are likely to be effectively targeted by concentrating on critical areas and by maximizing the chances of implementing change.

However, as with other approaches, there are some disadvantages.

- *Dissemination.* There is a danger that knowledge gleaned in one locality may not be effectively disseminated, leading to duplication of effort or continuance of bad practice.
- *Lack of expertise in quality techniques.* Whilst staff may be experts at what they do, they do not necessarily understand the skills and techniques required to carry out quality procedures.
- *Lack of strategic dimension.* The local ownership of such projects means that it is not possible to draw up a comprehensive strategic programme to assure quality in all the healthcare procedures within a particular hospital or region.

The strengths and weaknesses of each type of approach are summarized in Table 2.1.

In practice, a mixed model is the most effective. Locally controlled initiatives need senior management support and involvement. Top-down strategic programmes need practitioner involvement to inform decision making and increase the chance of implementing change (Fig. 2.2).

Table 2.1 Summary of approaches to quality

Top-down	Process accreditation	Bottom-up
Advantages		
Consistency	Cost-effectiveness	Local ownership
Strategic planning		Local expertise
Independent scrutiny	Independent scrutiny	Effective targeting
Disadvantages		
Complexity and cost	Consistency over merit	Dissemination
Practitioner resistance	Disincentive to improve	Lack of quality expertise
Data collection	Snapshot of sample	Lack of strategic dimension
Failure to implement good practice		
Focus upon ease of measurement		

2.4   QUALITY IN THE CURRENT UK HEALTHCARE CONTEXT

Although the context discussed here is the NHS, many of the issues raised are relevant to public health systems in other countries such as France or Canada.

The cost to the nation of a publicly funded health service is rising, whether it is measured in real cash terms or as a percentage of gross domestic product (see Fig. 2.3). This may be ascribed to a number of factors, including:

- the ageing population
- the increased sophistication of treatment, leading to increased cost
- the ability to keep patients alive who would previously have died.

The response of the government in the 1980s was to initiate a series of reforms, which are still being enacted at the time of writing. The aim of these reforms was principally to deal with the accelerating cost of healthcare. A key part of this policy was to shift emphasis away from treating ill people to keeping people

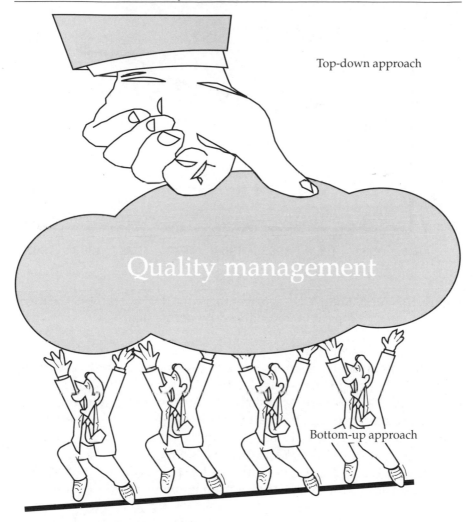

Top-down approach

Bottom-up approach

Figure 2.2   A mixed approach is generally best

healthy. This has the great benefit of being a 'good' thing both financially and from a health perspective.

The major health strategy is contained within the *Health of the Nation* document (DoH, 1992). This sets out targets in five key areas of health: CHD and stroke, cancer, mental illness, HIV/AIDS and sexual health, and accidents.

In strategic management terms, the 1992 White Paper is more akin to a mission statement than a strategy. It sets out aims,

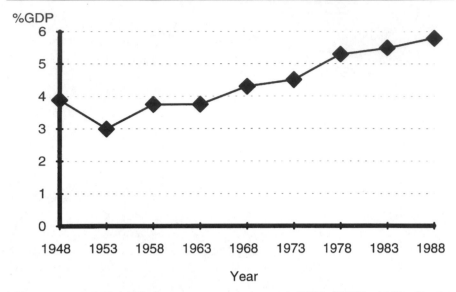

Figure 2.3 NHS budget as a percentage of GDP (OHE, 1989. Crown copyright, reproduced by permission)

objectives and targets in key areas. It contains limited information on implementation. In practice the key management structures were established in earlier legislation. However, the term 'structure' may be misleading as the management environment is characterized by continual change with mergers and demergers of health authorities: devolution to small units such as Hospital Trusts and fundholding GPs being reversed in some cases by merging of Trusts and the forming of GP consortia. One of the key characteristics of the NHS from a management point of view is its diversity.

Rather than taking a structural view of the service, this book will consider the organizational characteristics of the NHS over the period 1990–1995.

The Market

The key mechanism for introducing change into the NHS is the attempt to introduce 'market forces'. This process is not unique to the NHS: it has been the key instrument of change in the public sector as a whole.

The market has been introduced to the NHS by the establishment of 'purchasers' and 'suppliers'. The purchasers may be general practitioners directly if they have become fundholders and taken control of their own budgets, or alternatively Family Health Service Authorities may act upon behalf of other GPs. The suppliers are those providing services to the purchasers, usually Health Trusts, which may be hospitals, ambulance services or any other organization providing a service.

The market has been adopted with varying degrees of enthusiasm. In Lancashire, for example, at the end of 1994, only 21% of 170 GP practices were fundholding in spite of many inducements (Barrett et al, 1995).

Initially, the idea of independence was more attractive to hospitals, with the rate of 'opting out' and adoption of Trust status being much more rapid. All hospitals in Lancashire had become Trusts by 1993. However, this does not necessarily reflect any greater enthusiasm on the part of clinicians. The management structure of hospitals is much less clinically dominated than the management of general practices.

A number of Trusts are now experiencing difficulties and some are merging and forming larger units, which appears to run contrary to the initial trend.

In considering the market principle in the NHS we shall first consider the nature of the implementation in this context.

Competitive Forces

The issue is whether the NHS market has the same characteristics as a commercial market. The key characteristic of a market is the effect of competition. Company strategies are driven not so much by profit as by 'market share' and 'competitive advantage'. In simple terms, competition forces companies to be effective or to go to the wall.

This model simply does not transfer well to the public sector. No public sector body has actually been allowed to go bust. Where hospitals are shut or closure is attempted, closure is initiated by centralist intervention by the Secretary of State—the very opposite of market forces. Without this key competitive feature the market ideal can never be truly transferred.

The next feature required for competition to work is *choice*. In large urban conurbations, this is a realistic option: a general practitioner in Manchester has a range of hospitals to which to send patients. In a medium sized town (population ca. 150 000) it is unlikely that there is a realistic alternative to the local district hospital for the vast majority of clinical procedures.

A market cannot operate effectively where there is a virtual monopoly. Sometimes, in order to introduce a degree of competition, bizarre actions are taken. Recently, patients were shipped by ambulance over 200 miles to an under-used private facility that was offering very low prices to stave off receivership. Whilst this undoubtedly provided a benefit to the purchaser, the patients could argue that they were being manipulated for the benefit of the market rather than the other way around.

Who are the Customers?

Within any market situation, the effects of competition should ultimately be driven by the customer. Any introduction of an intermediary reduces the effectiveness of competition as an instrument of change. The role of customer in the NHS is a surprisingly ambiguous one. There are at least three significant 'customer' roles (Fig. 2.4).

The 'purchasers' are the direct customers in the NHS marketplace. They are the people and organizations with the power to effect change by placing their purchasing power elsewhere.

The patients might be considered the most obvious 'customers'

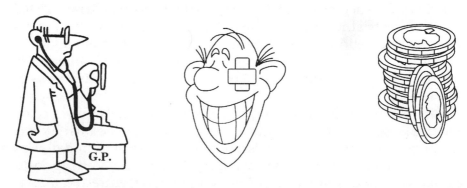

Figure 2.4   Who is the customer—NHS purchaser, patient, or purse holder?

of the NHS. However, they can only influence the market very marginally through their contact with purchasers. This clearly happens in a limited fashion. For example, in one local area there are two hospitals and about six consultants to whom a GP may refer an expectant mother. It is quite likely that the patient in this case will be able to influence the GP's choice of consultant and hospital. However, this influence is subject to a number of constraints. It is at the discretion of the GP and the hospital concerned. In cases where the mother wishes to adopt a less conventional approach, opting for a home birth and community midwife care throughout, the GP is much more likely to exercise his or her right to object. This may be right and proper from a clinical perspective, but it sets clear limits for the patient's ability to exercise choice as a customer.

The third customer role is the government through the Department of Health and the Treasury. The reforms were brought in to curb the spiralling costs of the National Health Service. As controller of the purse strings, the government is the ultimate customer with the power to use its purchasing power to influence the NHS market. Further, with the Department of Health reserving the right to go outside the market structure altogether in politically contentious areas, it may be seen as the real customer.

Price

The market is driven by competition and purchasing power is used to influence supplier behaviour. The next question is: which factors influence where purchasers place their custom?

The two key factors are price and quality of service. We shall return to quality later. For now let us simply concentrate on price. Purchasers have in theory a fixed budget with which to purchase healthcare for their patients. Therefore, they should be extremely sensitive to the price offered by suppliers, as they can get more treatment for the same money if they can get it cheaper.

Most of the problems to do with pricing actually arise at the supplier end. Hospitals have never before had to price their procedures accurately. Costs are very complex, involving both fixed and variable costs. Within a very short space of time hospitals were expected to be able to quote a cost for every clinical procedure they carried out.

This problem is not unique to the UK. In other countries, hospitals have faced similar problems. In Canada, a local health economist suggested that two approaches had been adopted. The first was a conscientious attempt to cost every procedure realistically. This almost inevitably seemed to produce an underestimate owing to failure to appreciate the true cost of factors such as depreciation. The alternative was described as sticking a finger in the air, i.e. making an intuitive guess. This actually proved more successful overall in the hospitals he had investigated, as the overestimates tended to cancel out the underestimates.

The problem of pricing has led to an unusual kind of contract. Suppliers agree to provide healthcare according to a contract which includes estimates of the cost. However, should these estimates prove to be wildly inaccurate, then the supplier may pass on the extra cost to the purchaser. This kind of agreement does tend to blunt the impact of price on purchaser behaviour. It also makes resource planning extremely difficult for both supplier and purchaser.

In fairness, this kind of contract is not unknown in other spheres. For example, large construction contracts often allow for time-scale and cost estimates to be renegotiated in the light of unforeseen contingencies. However, this is tightly controlled and is ultimately sanctioned by the purchaser, not the supplier.

In the light of these limitations upon the implementation of the market model, it is the author's view that the NHS market must be regarded as a 'pseudo-market'. We shall consider below the implications for quality assurance of the 'pseudo-market'.

The Division Between Clinicians and Managers

In order to implement the reforms, the impact of management upon the NHS has been increased. This has a number of consequences upon the culture of the organization. The mechanism of quality assurance has moved from a dependence upon the professionalism of individuals and groups to a formal quality assurance mechanism.

Clinicians have usually been offered a place in this management process. General practitioners have been offered the chance to manage their own budgets. Nurses have been offered a career progression structure leading to nursing management roles. In certain cases, management activities have been embraced enthusiastically by clinicians. For example, over 50% of clinical audits surveyed in the Oxford region were led by consultants (Ellis and Gillies, 1995).

However, in many other areas, clinicians and other healthcare professionals have not adopted a management role so enthusiastically. This may be for a number of reasons:

- a perception that they are there to treat patients, not manage
- resistance to change
- resistance to specific aspects of the reforms
- a perception of management as in opposition to professionalism
- fear that management will be used against them as individuals.

All of these reasons have been articulated by health professionals. The damaging consequence for the culture is a perceived divide between management activity and clinical activity. It is interesting to compare this reaction with other public sectors where management is accepted, if not willingly then grudgingly, such as in education. However, there are differences with education:

- Often NHS managers are not healthcare professionals, whereas education management is usually done by educators promoted to management grades.
- The education profession does not have strong central professional bodies and therefore has not been able to organize a centralized defence of 'professionalism'.
- The public has a much higher perception of the professionalism of doctors and nurses and is therefore more prepared to listen to arguments about the erosion of professionalism.

Whether professionalism and a managed health service are compatible or not, the cultural divide which often exists is detrimental to both professionalism and good management.

Further attempts to involve the clinical staff in management have often had the opposite effect, alienating staff further. One important difference between a 'management' view and a 'clinical' view is that managers are required to consider the needs of many people at once, whereas clinicians are required to do the best job they can for each and every patient. This can result in conflict where managers are interested in treating the highest number of patients in the shortest time at the least cost and clinicians wish to pay more attention to the needs of individual patients. This tends to make the managers look like the 'bad guys' and the clinicians the 'good guys' (Fig. 2.5).

What may represent good quality of care for an individual patient may result in another not seeing a doctor at all. This crucial dilemma between the needs of the many and the one is explored in more detail below.

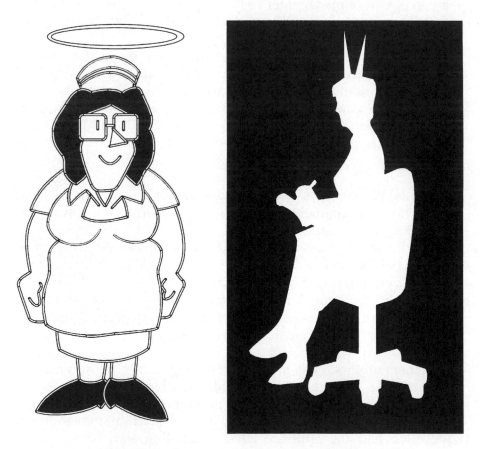

Figure 2.5 In practice, life is not so simple . . .

The Emphasis on Measurable Performance

One of the crucial elements of the NHS reforms is the emphasis on measured performance, allowing quantifiable improvements. In the words of Lord Kelvin:

Only when we can measure a problem can we understand it.

The 1992 White Paper *Health of the Nation* (DoH, 1992) establishes 27 targets all of which require measurement of performance. The two key questions which one may pose under this heading are:

• What can we measure?
• What effect does measurement have on the property to be measured?

Everybody likes quantifiable measures. Whilst the focus of the NHS was upon treating disease and illness, it was relatively easy to establish measurable parameters. Traditional measures include life expectancy, morbidity, and number of patients treated. Each of these is relatively easy to establish, and is broadly objective. However, health is a much more difficult thing to measure, because it is associated with quality of life rather than quantity. One is immediately in the realm of subjectivity, requiring indicators, rather than direct measurement. To establish the difference, consider the difference between:

• How many patients survived?
• How many patients made a full recovery?

The first question simply requires the subtraction of the number of patients who died from the total number treated. The second requires all sorts of subjective judgements about a 'full recovery' and indicators of it.

Consider another deceptively simple measure, the number of pregnancies resulting from an IVF programme. This begs the question of what a successful pregnancy is. Is it:

(a) fertilization?

(b)   establishment of a viable foetus within the womb?
(c)   a foetus reaching the level of development detectable by a pregnancy test?
(d)   carrying the baby to full term?
(e)   a live birth?
(f)   a healthy child free from genetic defects?

Equally contentious are measures of performance in areas such as waiting time. Is the waiting time for an appointment, the time from seeing your GP to seeing the hospital doctor, or from when you enter the hospital's appointment system? Is it acceptable to trade waiting times for an appointment for waiting times at the clinic by cramming in more patients to each clinic to reduce waiting lists?

The key issue here is that each of these indicators shows only part of an overall picture. By quoting a single indicator you can present the view of the situation that is most advantageous or disadvantageous dependent upon which axe you wish to grind.

Performance is always a multidimensional construct and it is always constrained. We can use two pictures to illustrate this. Consider performance as a polyhedron, a cube for ease of drawing, as shown in Fig. 2.6. You can never see all the sides of a

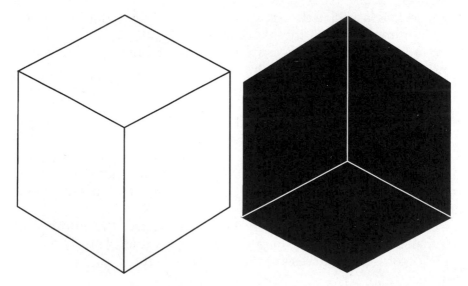

Figure 2.6   Three sides of the cube are not the whole picture

polyhedron at once. If you quote only the fact that the cube is white from seeing three sides (the left picture) you may miss the fact that the other three faces are black. If the performance here is the 'blackness' of the cube, then looking at the three white faces would give you a performance of zero. Looking at the black faces gives you a figure of 100%. An average, if measured as a mean, would imply a uniform greyness or 50% blackness. Only by considering each aspect or face of the cube can we actually give a true representation.

The other aspect is that performance is subject to constraints. There are internal constraints, since each aspect is likely to be dependent upon the others. Thus, we can reduce the waiting time for an appointment at the clinic by increasing the number of patients per clinic and therefore increasing the waiting time at the clinic itself. This may be visualized as a half-inflated balloon being squashed: as we squash it in one place it simply expands some-where else (Fig. 2.7).

To relieve the internal constraints we must remove the external constraints which are usually resource-based. Thus if we put more resources into our clinic, we can see more patients without

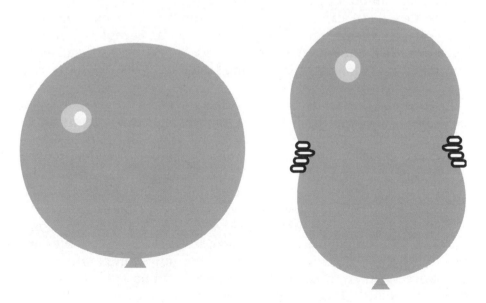

Figure 2.7   Quality is constrained

increasing the waiting time at the clinic itself. However, as the overall resource level is finite, this merely leads to less resources elsewhere in the service.

Lord Kelvin's quotation was from the field of physics where objectivity is often easier to achieve. However, quantum physics can lend us another insight which we should note when considering the measurement of performance. Heisenburg's Uncertainty Principle states that the observation of an effect perturbs the effect itself. Thus as soon as we try to observe the precise location of an object we in fact disturb its position. However, this is a quantum effect operating at subatomic levels and distances of less than 10^{-10} metres.

There is however a macroscopic analogue of this effect. If you tell a group of practitioners that they will be measured on a particular aspect of their performance they will naturally concentrate their efforts in that area. Thus if you tell someone that success is to be measured in terms of the smallness of the horizontal diameter of a balloon, they squeeze it at the sides. If you tell them that it will be measured as the vertical diameter, they squeeze it at the top and bottom. Thus performance measurement can distort performance.

A certain amount of this is desirable as part of the prioritization of resources. But care is needed. Measures can be manipulated. Thus, if you wish to measure patients seen as completed patient episodes, then patients may be referred on to other specialists to complete the patient episode and referred back to the same consultant as a 'new' patient.

In extremis, hospitals appear to have written to patients who have been on a waiting list for 11 months and taken them off to prevent them waiting more than 12 months. The patient is re-registered shortly afterwards and the hospital reduces the number of patients waiting more than 12 months at least in terms of the way that the performance is measured. To misquote Disraeli: 'There are lies, damned lies and performance indicators ...'.

The final contentious area considered here is the use of comparative measurement to produce league tables. League tables are produced these days which purport to show comparative performance in many areas of almost every public service. All the problems raised above apply to comparative measurement. Two further issues are introduced:

- the issue of 'added value'
- the 'nothing sacred' issue.

The first issue has been raised most prominently in the area of education, but applies equally to medicine. Consider a GP in a suburban area. His performance in health screening is measured and he is near the top of the league. Compare his colleague in the inner city. Her performance is poor and she is placed near the bottom of the league. Who is more successful? The first doctor has women demanding smears annually rather than the recommended three-year frequency. The second has a very mobile population to serve with a rapid turnover of patients. The patients are generally poor, anxious about authority, have reading difficulties in many cases and are much harder to reach. Raw performance indicators will not reveal the effectiveness of either doctor in reaching their target population.

The second issue was raised recently when a doctor mooted the possibility of having to provide league tables of infertility clinics measured according to their success rates in achieving pregnancies. In matters such as this, performance measurement has explicit ethical implications.

The next chapter develops models of quality to deal with some of the issues raised in this chapter in more detail.

2.5   REFERENCES

Barrett, M. et al (1995) IT and IS in general practice. *Proceedings of the First International Symposium on Health Information Management Research, Sheffield, 5–7 April*, 112–118.

Cohen, I. B. (1984) Florence Nightingale. *Scientific American*, (250), 98–107.

Crombie, I. K., Davies, H. T. O., Abraham, S. C. S. & du V. Florey, C. (1993) *The Audit Handbook: Improving Healthcare Through Clinical Audit*. Chichester: Wiley.

Department of Health (1992) *The Quality of Medical Care: Report of the Standing Medical Advisory Committee*. London: HMSO.

Ellis, N. T. & Gillies, A. C. (1995) The reality of medical audit: the Oxford experience. *Proceedings of the First International Symposium on Health Information Management Research, Sheffield, 5–7 April*, 34–43.

Godber, G. (1976) The confidential enquiry into maternal deaths. In:

McLaughlin, G. A. (ed.), *A Question of Quality*. London: Oxford University Press, 24–33.

Jonas, S. & Rosenberg, S. N. (1986) Measurement and control in the quality of health care. In: Jonas, S. (ed.), *Health Care Delivery in the United States*. New York: Springer Verlag, 416–64.

Lembcke, P. A. (1967) Evolution of the medical audit. *Journal of the American Medical Association*, **199**, 111–18.

Office of Health Economics (1989) *Compendium of Health Statistics*. London: HMSO.

Roberts, J. S., Coale, J. G. & Redman, R. R. (1987) A history of the Joint Commission of the Accreditation of Hospitals. *Journal of the American Medical Association*, **258**, 936–40.

Smith, C. W. (1950) *Florence Nightingale*. London: Constable.

CHAPTER 3

Measuring Quality

3.1 CHAPTER SUMMARY

This chapter introduces the idea of modelling quality. Most of the models used are hierarchical in nature. Hierarchical models are introduced in general terms first, using a school example. Such models divide quality into distinct criteria and then seek to measure quality under each criteria.

A detailed hierarchical model of primary health care is demonstrated, drawn from the Management Advancement Program (MAP) developed by the Aga Khan Foundation and promoted by the World Health Organization.

The chapter discusses the problem of measurement through the use of indicators. Indicators are divided according to whether they measure inputs, outputs or effects. The text argues that effect indicators are the most useful but the most difficult to measure; input indicators are easier to measure but are less informative. Sample indicators are discussed for parts of the MAP and used to demonstrate the characteristics of the different indicator types.

Finally, the problem of representing overall quality using a hierarchical scheme is discussed. Numerical schemes are described but all share the disadvantage of a loss of information content in the collation process. Graphical schemes are preferable. The text argues for the benefits of the humble bar chart. It goes on to discuss some more complex graphical devices, but points out some of the potential pitfalls.

3.2   HIERARCHICAL MODELS OF QUALITY

In order to compare quality in different situations, both qualitatively and quantitatively, it is necessary to establish a model of quality. Many models have been suggested, most of them hierarchical in nature. In order to examine the nature of hierarchical models, consider the methods of assessment and reporting used in schools. The progress of a particular student has generally been recorded under a series of headings, usually subject areas such as Science, English, Maths and Humanities (Fig. 3.1).

A qualitative assessment is generally made, along with a more quantified assessment. These measures may be derived from a formal test or examination, continuous assessment of coursework or a quantified teacher assessment. In practice, the resulting scores are derived from a whole spectrum of techniques. They range from those which may be regarded as objective and transferable, to those which are simply a more convenient representation of

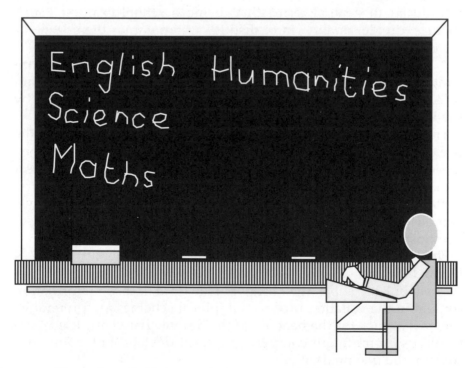

Figure 3.1   Student 'quality' is assessed under subject areas

qualitative judgements. In the past, these have been gathered together to form a traditional school report (Table 3.1).

The traditional school report often had an overall mark and grade—a single figure, generally derived from the mean of the component figures, intended to provide a single measure of success.

In recent years, the assessment of pupils has become considerably more sophisticated and the model on which the assessment is based has become more complicated. Subjects are now broken down into skills, each of which is measured and the collective results used to give a more detailed overall picture. For example, in English, pupils' oral skills are considered alongside their ability to read; written English is further sub-divided into an assessment of style, content and presentation. The hierarchical model requires another level of sophistication in order to accommodate the changes (Fig. 3.2).

Much effort is currently being devoted to producing a broader based assessment, and in ensuring that qualitative judgements are as accurate and consistent as possible. The aim is for every pupil to emerge with a broad-based 'Record of Achievement' alongside their more traditional examination results.

Many of the points raised within the context of pupil assessment are paralleled in the assessment of the quality of healthcare. A similar hierarchical approach, considering quality under a series of headings, is adopted by many authors. The resulting models are therefore known as hierarchical models. A hierarchical model of quality is based upon a set of quality criteria, each of which has

Table 3.1 A traditional school report

Subject	Teacher's comments	Term grade (A ... E)	Exam mark (%)
English			
Maths			
Science			
Humanities			
Languages			
Technology			
OVERALL			

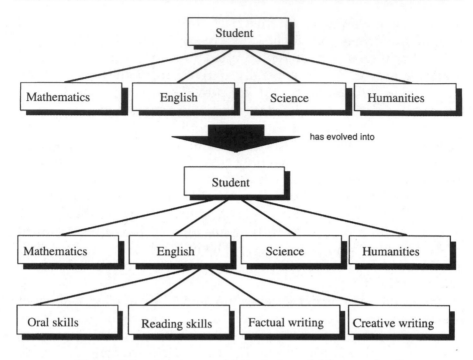

Figure 3.2   A more sophisticated model has evolved

a set of measures or indicators associated with it. This type of model is illustrated schematically in Fig. 3.3.

3.3   A HIERARCHICAL MODEL OF PRIMARY HEALTHCARE

A hierarchical model of the quality of primary healthcare has been described by Franco et al (1993). The overall framework of the model is shown in Fig. 3.4.

Within this model, the quality of primary healthcare is considered under five headings:

- the quality of general care
- the quality of maternity care
- the quality of child care
- the quality of community healthcare
- the quality of other primary care.

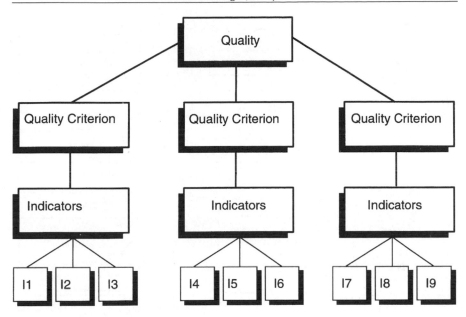

Figure 3.3 A hierarchical model of quality (schematic)

Nineteen criteria of care are defined to cover these five categories. In order to complete such a model it is necessary to provide a method to measure performance under each of these criteria.

3.4   THE PROBLEM OF MEASUREMENT

Quality measurement, where it is considered at all, is usually expressed in terms of indicators. An indicator is a measurable property that varies in accordance with the quality criteria that we are seeking to measure. As such, there are a number of conditions that a performance indicator must meet. It must:

- be clearly linked to the quality criterion that it seeks to measure
- be sensitive to the different degrees of the criterion
- provide objective determination of the criterion that can be mapped on to a suitable scale.

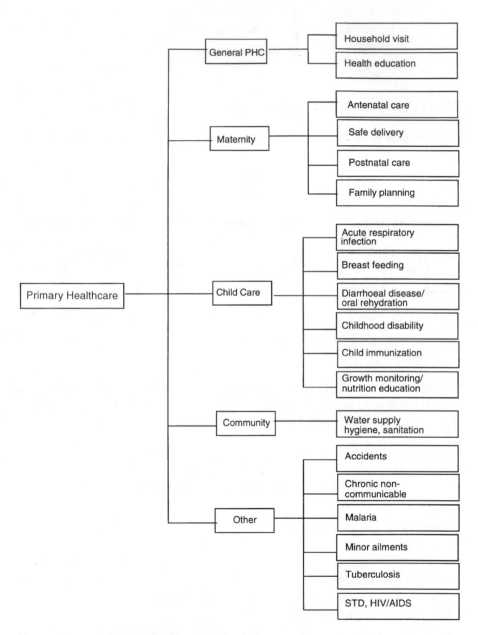

Figure 3.4   A hierarchical model of the quality of primary healthcare delivery

However, indicators are not the same as direct measures. Consider the traditional fairground trial of strength (Fig. 3.5). It does not measure strength in a direct, absolute and verifiable way, but rather gives an indication of strength in terms of the height reached up the column. The height reached is proportional to the force exerted upon the plate at the bottom, but this is affected by factors other than strength, such as swing technique. The height attained is, therefore, like a metric of strength, i.e. a measurable property which is related to the criteria under investigation. We must establish that the metric (height) provides an accurate representation of the measurable property (force exerted upon the plate), which in turn should correlate well with the actual property under investigation (strength). Social scientists are comfortable in dealing with messy multivariate problems. Engineers and scientists are often less so. Doctors have generally been

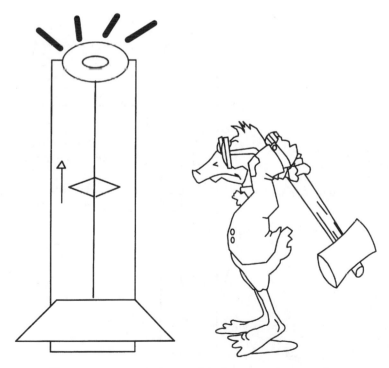

Figure 3.5 A traditional indicator of strength

trained within a scientific paradigm and therefore may not be comfortable with such problems, although clinical diagnosis is often an extremely fuzzy problem.

Contrast the fairground scenario with taking the temperature of a patient. This uses the expansion of mercury to measure temperature (Fig. 3.6). The relationship between linear expansion and temperature rise is direct, linear and verifiable by experiment. Expansion depends only upon temperature, and calibration points exist at the freezing and boiling points of water to establish an absolute scale.

Quality criteria are never dependent upon a single property in this way and no reference points exist to establish an absolute scale. Many people find it difficult to adjust to consideration of the quality of health care delivered, which cannot be measured in terms of simple, absolute and unambiguous scales. In the next section we shall see how indicators may be used to measure quality within the hierarchical model described above.

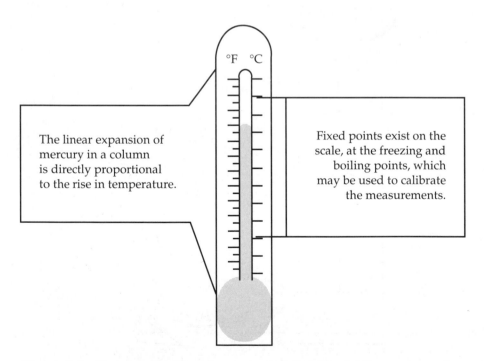

The linear expansion of mercury in a column is directly proportional to the rise in temperature.

°F °C

Fixed points exist on the scale, at the freezing and boiling points, which may be used to calibrate the measurements.

Figure 3.6   Temperature may be measured in terms of linear expansion

3.5   USING PERFORMANCE INDICATORS TO MEASURE PRIMARY HEALTHCARE PERFORMANCE

Within the framework described by Franco et al (1993), each of the 19 criteria may be measured in terms of an indicator of effect, output or input. In general terms, indicators of effect are more useful than those of output which are in turn are more useful than those of inputs. However, the ease of collection of information is often in inverse proportion to the usefulness of the measurement.

Table 3.2 summarizes indicators for general care, health education and antenatal care.

Another way of classifying indicators is in terms of the different views of the stakeholders in the healthcare process. Chapter 1 identified five views of the quality of healthcare based upon a Garvin-style model: the transcendent view; the public health view; the resource-based view; the professional view; and the patient-based view. One of the difficulties of the transcendent view of quality is that it cannot easily be measured. In practice, it may be represented as the collation of the other views, or as a hierarchy as shown in Fig. 3.7.

We may consider indicators according to which view they represent. This is important because different stakeholders will often quote specific and isolated indicators in order to emphasize a particular viewpoint. Table 3.3 provides examples of indicators according to the views that they represent.

It may also be seen that different views lend themselves to different types of indicators. For example, a resource-based view of quality naturally favours input indicators, since resources are themselves an input. Other views such as the patient-based view reflect that patients are concerned with effective treatment and only consider inputs and outputs as far as they impact upon the effect.

The public health view reflects the time lag that often exists between being able to measure inputs and effects. In public health programmes, screening or education programmes are introduced. Initially, quality may be judged by the size and extent of the screening programme. This is an input indicator. The next indicator is the percentage of the target population reached by the programme. This is an output indicator. Finally, after what is often a considerable time the effect may be judged by gathering

Table 3.2 Illustrative indicators of healthcare provision

Criteria	Type	Indicators
Household visits	Output	% households visited in last 3 months % households visited in last 3 months where specific topic discussed, e.g. family planning % households visited in last 3 months by type, e.g. age or risk
	Input	Households per health worker Population per health worker Number of health workers by type, e.g. community nurse, midwife
	Effect	% respondents who show behaviour in accordance with objectives % respondents who remember broadcast health messages % respondents who remember message from last visit
Health education	Output	% of target population visited within last 3 months % health workers using 1 or more health education techniques % of target population receiving health information in a group
	Input	% of health workers trained in health education % of community organizations providing health information Health workers per 1000 households

Antenatal care	Effect	% of target population wishing to receive further information
	Output	% of women receiving at least one antenatal visit
		Mean number of contacts per pregnant woman
		% of women seen counselled about danger signs
		% of workers tracking high risk pregnancies
		% of high risk women seen by health worker identified as such
		% of workers providing medical attention to high risk pregnancies
	Input	% health units experiencing shortages of supplements
		No of days for which supplements were out of stock at clinic
		% of women of reproductive age weighing $<38\mathrm{Kg}$ before pregnancy
	Effect	% of pregnant women identified as high risk
		% of women making 3 or more antenatal visits during their last pregnancy
		% of women receiving two doses of tetanus
		% of women complying with iron folate supplements programme
		% of women gaining $<1\,\mathrm{kg}$ during 2nd and 3rd trimester

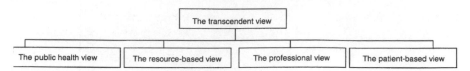

Figure 3.7   Views of quality expressed as a hierarchical model

Table 3.3   Indicators classified according to the view that they represent

View	Type	Sample indicator
Public health	Effect	% of target teenage population becoming pregnant
	Output	Number of condoms distributed to target population
	Input	% of teenagers with access to family planning clinics
Resource-based	Effect	Morbidity amongst target population per £000 spent
	Output	Number of patient episodes per pound
	Input	Departmental annual budget
Professional	Effect	Number of patient episodes judged to be clinically successful
	Output	Number of patient episodes
	Input	Number of clinicians
Patient-based	Effect	Waiting time to be free of illness
	Output	Waiting time for appointment
	Input	Distance to nearest hospital

information on public health issues, such as teenage pregnancy rates, or cancer morbidity data.

The objective measurement of quality through the use of indicators within a hierarchical framework is an attractive one. However, the indicators available are limited in effectiveness for a whole series of reasons. These will be considered in the next section.

3.6   THE PROBLEMS WITH INDICATORS

They cannot be validated.   As mentioned above, the relationships between the indicators and the criteria that they seek to measure are complex. It is difficult to establish the degree of correlation between the indicator itself, the measurable upon which it is based, and the criteria which it seeks to measure. As might be imagined, it is harder still to validate the degree of correlation.

They are not generally objective.   In an ideal world, measures would be objective, absolute and transferable. In practice, all measures are relative, but the presence of 'fixed points', (e.g. absolute zero and the triple point of water on the temperature scale) allow some scales to be defined as effectively absolute, and hence transferable and objective. In quality, there are no fixed points. Some measures may appear to be transferable and objective, such as measures based upon waiting times for appointments. However, such objective figures generally refer to inputs rather than effects. Further, they may be used for comparison when they are not comparable.

Quality is a relative, not an absolute, quantity.   In practice, many aspects of quality can only be judged in relative terms. For example, it is hard to imagine ever establishing an absolute reference point for health. Health can only be measured relative to other experiences. What may be described as healthy in one patient in one situation may be considered unhealthy in another.

The criteria of quality and their indicators are not independent.   A major limitation of hierarchical models is that they assume that overall quality of healthcare can be neatly partitioned into a series of criteria. This is simply not the case. Criteria show complex interrelationships, and in reality, overall quality is more than the sum of the parts.

So far it has been assumed that if we can measure the individual quality criteria, then we can derive a measure of total quality. This is considered in the next section.

3.7   AN OVERALL MEASURE OF QUALITY

Much of the work in this area has been concerned with simple reduction of a set of scores to a single 'figure-of-merit'. There are a number of possible approaches, most of which have been used at one time or another in quality management.

Simple Scoring

In this method, each criterion is allocated a score. The overall quality is given by the mean of the individual scores.

Weighted Scoring

This scheme allows the user to weight each criterion according to how important they consider it to be. This approach is compared with simple scoring in Table 3.4.

Each criterion is evaluated to produce a percentage. In the case of simple scoring the scores are added and divided by the number of scores to yield a simple arithmetic mean. In the weighted case, each score is weighted before summation and the resulting figure reflects the relative importance of the different factors. The result obtained by simple scoring is thus given by:

$$\text{Simple Score} = 685/9 = 76\%.$$

The weighted score, giving in general more weight to effect indicators, is given by:

$$\text{Weighted Score} = 320.5/4.3 = 74.5\%.$$

Table 3.4   Examples of simple and weighted scoring methods

Indicator	Type	Raw score	Weight	Product
Number of clinics per week/ target (%)	Input	90	0.3	27
Number of doctors per clinic/ target (%)	Input	90	0.2	18
% of time scan facilities available	Input	70	0.1	7
Number of patients seen per week/target (%)	Output	85	0.5	42.5
% utilization of available appointments	Output	70	0.4	28
% of patients requiring scans	Output	65	0.4	26
% of patients correctly treated	Effect	90	0.8	72
% of patients treated before complications	Effect	50	0.8	40
% of patients not returning within 3 yrs	Effect	75	0.8	60
TOTALS		685	4.3	320.5

Phased Weighting Factor Method

This is an extension of weighted scoring. In this method, a weighting is assigned to a group of characteristics before each individual weighting is considered. If we apply the same weighting as to the previous case, but with an additional weighting of $\frac{1}{2}$ for those indicators reflecting effects, $\frac{1}{4}$ for those indicators reflecting outputs and $\frac{1}{4}$ for those indicators reflecting inputs, then the result is as illustrated in Table 3.5.

The mean of the input scores is 83.3%.

The mean of the output scores is 73.3%.

The mean of the effect scores is 71.7%.

Table 3.5 The phased weighting factor method

Indicator	Type	Raw score	Weight	Product	PWF
Number of clinics per week/target (%)	Input	90	0.3	27	$\frac{1}{4}$
Number of doctors per clinic/target (%)	Input	90	0.2	18	$\frac{1}{4}$
% of time scan facilities available	Input	70	0.1	7	$\frac{1}{4}$
Number of patients seen per week/ target (%)	Output	85	0.5	42.5	$\frac{1}{4}$
% utilization of available appointments	Output	70	0.4	28	$\frac{1}{4}$
% of patients requiring scans	Output	65	0.4	26	$\frac{1}{4}$
% of patients correctly treated	Effect	90	0.8	72	$\frac{1}{2}$
% of patients treated before complications	Effect	50	0.8	40	$\frac{1}{2}$
% of patients not returning within 3 yrs	Effect	75	0.8	60	$\frac{1}{2}$
TOTALS		685	4.3	320.5	

The overall phased weighted scoring value is given by:

$$PWF = \tfrac{1}{4}(83.3\%) + \tfrac{1}{4}(73.3\%) + \tfrac{1}{2}(71.7\%) = 75\%.$$

Each of these schemes is aimed at reducing the quality measure to a single parameter. The biggest problem with this approach is that in order to obtain a single figure, the level of information has reduced to a level which is completely unhelpful.

An alternative approach is to use graphical profiles to maintain the information content whilst presenting a multidimensional view of quality.

3.8   GRAPHICAL QUALITY PROFILES

If we consider the example above then it may be represented simply as a bar chart (Fig. 3.8). The use of simple graphs which display performance as a percentage of the target may be over-looked because of its simplicity. However, simple techniques are usually best in visual representation. We shall consider one alternative, the plotting of indicators around a circular chart.

Circular Charts

The use of circular graphical techniques in profiles was pioneered by Kostick as part of the proprietary PAPI technique used by PA management consultants for personnel profiling. The wider use of such graphs has been suggested by the author for image quality (Gillies, 1990). The graphs are particularly useful for the communication and comparison of multivariate properties such as a personnel profile or software quality. Within personnel profiling,

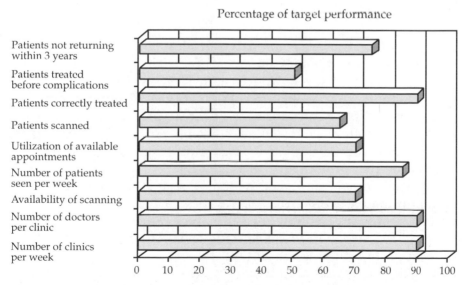

Figure 3.8   Displaying overall quality of healthcare delivered as a simple graph

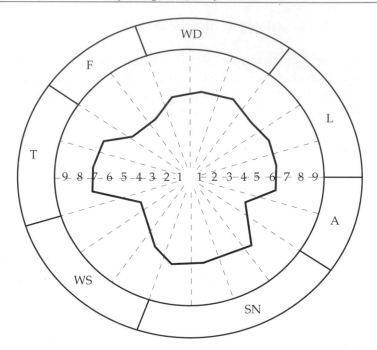

Figure 3.9 Schematic PAPI profile: WD = work direction, L = leader-ship, A = activity, SN = social nature, WS = work style, T = tempera-ment, F = followership

the technique is based upon a questionnaire, from which 20 personality characteristics are measured. The characteristics are then gathered into seven groups, namely Work Direction, Leadership, Activity, Social Nature, Work Style, Temperament and Followership. The scores for each of the 20 profiles, in the range 1 to 9, are plotted on a circular graph, using a linear scale, producing a profile (Fig. 3.9). These profiles may then compared with each other or with an 'ideal' template.

This technique is employed within personnel management when trying to match people to a job vacancy or task. The profile does not relate to any overall measure, but rather to the blend of characteristics required for a specific task. As such, it is the shape of the profile that is important rather than the overall area enclosed. The graphs are popular because of their ease of use and comparison, and because of their ability to display multiple data as a single shape.

Radar Charts

Suitable graphical techniques should allow the multidimensionality of quality to be retained, whilst providing an overall impression of quality. The author has made use of such graphs for displaying image quality. A related technique is the radar chart utilized in some quality assurance procedures. A radar chart based upon the sample data given in Table 3.5 is shown in Fig. 3.10.

Radar charts are used quite extensively in quality management applications to display quality data. However, they can actually provide a misleading view of the overall situation.

An important distinction between Kostick graphs and radar charts is that Kostick charts do not assign any significance to the area contained by the profile. Radar charts do, however, and so the link between the area and the individual scores must be established. It is by no means a simple linear relationship.

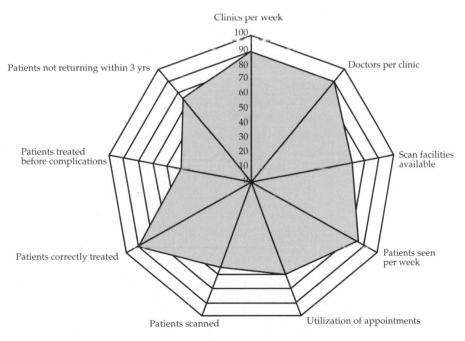

Figure 3.10 Radar chart based upon data in Table 3.5

Factors Affecting the Area in the Radar Chart

The factors affecting the area, other than the contributing values of the indicators displayed, are:

- the linear scale
- the division of the circle
- the neighbour effect.

The Radial Scale

Radar charts in theory permit the plotting of an infinite number of dimensions around the circle. However, the profile is made up of a series of triangles and the whole area is given by the sum of the areas of these:

$$\text{Area} = \sum_{i=1}^{i=n} \tfrac{1}{2} x_i x_{i-1} \sin\left[(\theta_i + \theta_{i+1})/2\right]. \qquad (3.1)$$

This means that, overall, the area contained is proportional to x^2, not x. A better method would therefore be to plot the square roots of the values. The effect of this on the above plot is shown in Fig. 3.11.

Division of the Circle

Input indicators are the easiest to measure, but effect indicators are the most useful. Since input indicators are the easiest to measure, there are often more of these available. Simply to take account equally of all available indicators would lead to domination by those characteristics which are most easily measured. In practice, this often happens in quality assessment. See for example the author's work on software quality (Gillies, 1996).

It is therefore necessary to decide the relative weights of input, output and effect indicators. In qualitative terms, it may be stated that effects are more important than outputs, which are more important than inputs. Therefore, a 3:2:1 weighting may be considered as reasonable. This may be viewed as the graphical analogue of the phased weighting factor method discussed above.

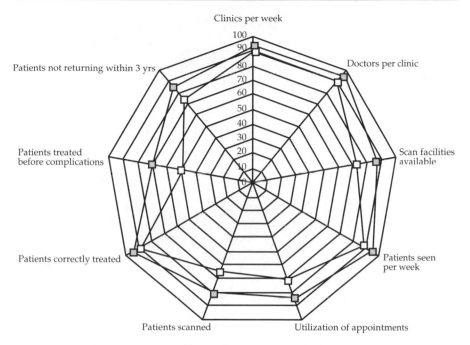

Figure 3.11 Effect of using a square-root scale

The effect of this upon the previous profile is illustrated in Fig. 3.12, using the square root of the indicator scores.

In cases where there are more indicators provided for one category than another, then the relative areas are determined by the overall weighting, not simply the number of indicators. Thus if we consider a modified version of the above example where the indicator for patients not returning is unavailable but an additional input indicator for the annual departmental budget is included, then the chart resulting is shown in Fig. 3.13.

The Neighbour Effect

It may also be seen from Eqn 3.1 that the area depends not simply upon the individual scores, but upon the sum of the products of the adjacent scores. This means that the area will be sensitive to the ordering of the characteristics around the graph, which is undesirable.

To illustrate the effects described, the data set used to calculate

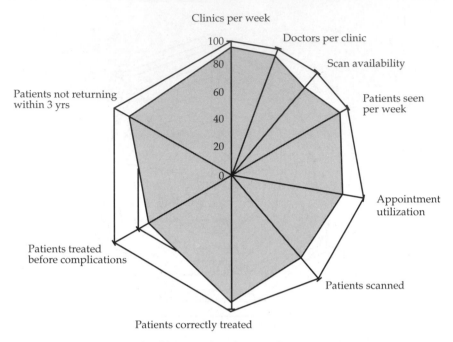

Figure 3.12   Profile weighted according to indicator type

the graph in Fig. 3.13 will be compared with a data set where all the indicator values are precisely half. Two sets of data will be used to calculate actual differences arising from each of the factors mentioned above. The second set is derived from the first. Each value is simply half that in the first set. The test data are shown in Table 3.6.

Using a spreadsheet, the area enclosed was calculated for a number of cases:

(a) linear scale/indicators given equal weighting (as per PAPI)
(b) linear scale/indicator types given equal weighting
(c) root scale/indicators given equal weighting
(d) root scale/indicator types given equal weighting
(e) root scale/indicator types given 3:2:1 weighting.

The resulting areas representing an indicator of total quality are shown in Table 3.7.

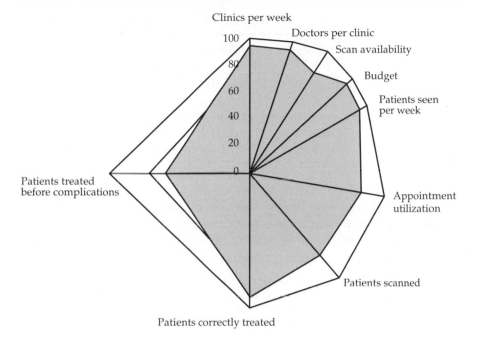

Figure 3.13 Example with more input indicators

Table 3.6 Sample data sets used to demonstrate effects

Indicator	Dataset1		Dataset2	
	Raw %	*Root %*	*Raw %*	*Root %*
Clinics per week	90	94.9	45	67.1
Doctors per clinic	90	94.9	45	67.1
Scan availability	70	83.7	35	59.2
Budget	95	97.5	47.5	68.9
Patients seen per week	85	92.2	42.5	65.2
Utilization of appointments	70	83.7	35	59.2
Patients scanned	65	80.6	32.5	57.0
Patients correctly treated	90	94.9	45	67.1
Patients treated before complications	50	70.7	25	50.0

Table 3.7   Areas enclosed by different profiling schemes

Case	Scale	Weighting by	Type	Area1	Area2	Ratio
1	Linear	Indicator	Equal	1.751	0.438	4
2	Linear	Ind. type	Equal	1.643	0.411	4
3	Root	Indicator	Equal	2.237	1.118	2
4	Root	Ind. type	Equal	2.069	1.034	2
5	Root	Ind. type	3:2:1	1.703	0.851	2

These examples show that unless a root scale is used, a doubling of scores leads to a quadrupling of the area.

However, it is also possible to show that, since the overall area depends upon the difference between adjacent values, then by changing the order of the graph the area enclosed changes. If we allow the ordering within each indicator type to vary, then using a linear scale, the area can vary between 1.68 and 1.78.

Table 3.8 shows the ordering of indicators required to enclose the minimum and maximum areas.

Removal of the Ordering Effect

The effect of neighbours is not a severe problem in schemes such as PAPI, where the overall area is not assessed quantitatively and

Table 3.8   Ordering of indicators

Minimum area enclosed by:	Maximum area enclosed by:
Scan availability	Budget
Clinics per week	Clinics per week
Doctors per clinic	Scan availability
Budget	Doctors per clinic
Patients seen per week	Patients scanned
Utilization of appointments	Patients seen per week
Patients scanned	Utilization of appointments
Patients correctly treated	Patients treated before complications
Patients treated before complications	Patients correctly treated

the order of the parameters does not change. However, where the area is intended to give an overall measure of quality, and the parameters themselves may vary, it is essential to make the area independent of the order in which the parameters are plotted. This cannot be achieved whilst the area of each segment depends upon the adjacent values. This means that the current connected polygon must be abandoned if the scheme is to be made independent of the ordering.

An alternative procedure is to include rules for ordering of profiles in a model which can be used as a basis for conventional charts. Two schemes are proposed, one which strives for maximum rigour, the other which seeks to retain the current radar chart format.

A Constant Area Profile Graph

The circular format is retained, with a radial scale. However, the scale runs from the outside into the centre. The profile is plotted from the circumference to the profile points and back between each point. In this fashion, the area depends principally upon the value plotted. A typical profile of this type, based upon the first data set in Table 3.6, is shown in Fig. 3.14.

The area of each section may be determined as follows. Consider the profile component shown in Fig. 3.15. If we let the angle defined at the centre by the sector OPQR be θ, then the area of quadrilateral OPQR is given by:

$$\text{Quadrilateral OPQR} = r^2 \sin(\theta/2). \tag{3.2}$$

The area of the corresponding sector is given by:

$$\text{Area of Sector OPQR} = \pi r^2(\theta_i/2\pi) = r^2\theta_i/2. \tag{3.3}$$

For small θ_i, $\theta_i \sim \sin\theta_i$, and then:

$$\text{Area of Sector} \sim \text{Area of Quadrilateral OPQR}.$$

The significance of this for the constant area profile is that it should be defined in terms of quadrilateral sections rather than sectors. The area of the quadrilateral profile section (OPQR) is

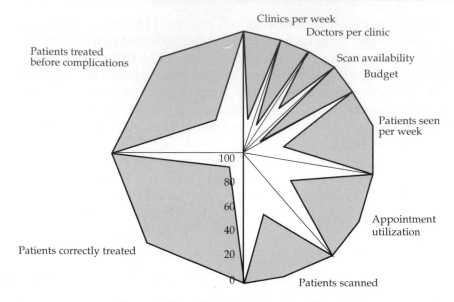

Figure 3.14 Constant area profile graph

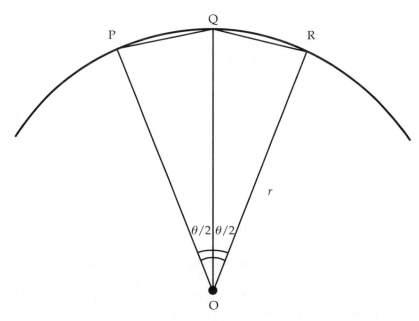

Figure 3.15 Terms used in text

given by Eqn 3.2 for all values of θ_i, whereas the area of the sector is proportional to the sine of the angle. This means that if we define our measures on a scale from zero to 1, setting r equal to 1, the area contained by the whole profile depends upon the measure and the sine of the angle symbol $\theta_i/2$

If the indicator types are represented by differing numbers of indicators, then in order to maintain consistent contributions from different characteristics with different numbers of measures, it is necessary to apply a factor which corrects for the dependency upon the number of measures, which determines the angle $\theta_i/2$:

$$\text{Plotted Value} = \text{Measured Value} \times \text{Correction Factor} \qquad (3.4)$$

where

$$\text{Correction Factor} = \frac{(\theta_i/2)}{\sin(\theta_i/2)} \qquad (3.5)$$

and $\theta_i = (\pi/2) \times (1/\text{number of characteristics}) \times (1/\text{number of measures})$.

If the different indicator types are to be weighted, then this should be incorporated into the correction factor:

$$\text{Weighted Correction Factor} = \text{Type Weighting} \times \text{Correction Factor}$$
$$(3.6)$$

where the type weighting is 1 for input indicators, 2 for output indicators, and 3 for effect indicators. The weighted correction factor is then normalized with respect to the maximum correction factor:

$$\text{Scaled Correction Factor} = \frac{\text{Weighted Correction Factor}}{\text{Maximum Correction Factor}}. \qquad (3.7)$$

Plotted in this manner, our profile has the following properties:

(1) The area of the profile depends linearly upon the values.
(2) The area of the profile is independent of the order of measures.
(3) The area is not affected by the number of indicators, only by

the weighting ascribed to each type if a type weighting factor is used.

Radar Charts Based Upon an Internal Model to Minimize Distortions

The above approach is rigorous but suffers from complexity and from the fact that the area contained is not a continuous polygon. For these reasons, it may prove unattractive.

The more common radar charts may be used with some modifications and provide a good indication of overall quality if the following procedures are observed.

(a) The data plotted must be the square root of the actual measures.
(b) The division of the area should be by indicator type, not the number of individual measures available. Division may be equal or weighted.
(c) The simplest approach is to say that each type of indicator be allocated an equal contribution by using the same number of input, output and effect indicators. This is the only approach which may be used with a conventional radar chart and is shown in Fig. 3.11.
(d) Given that effect indicators generally tell us far more about quality than outputs or inputs, the 3:2:1 weighting rule which weights the allocation of area in favour of effects and outputs seems to be the most informative. An example of this type is shown in Fig. 3.13.
(e) In order to minimize the effect of ordering, the following rules should be applied:
   – Indicators should be grouped into types and then plotted in the order: inputs, then outputs, then effects in a clockwise direction.
   – Within types, indicators should be plotted in ascending order, unless the order has been fixed previously in an earlier or comparative study where changing the order will prevent comparison.

Used in this way, radar charts can provide a useful view of overall performance.

3.9 REFERENCES

Franco, L. M., Richardson, P., Reynolds, J. & Meeraj, K. (1993) *Management Advancement Program Vol. 5: Performance Indicators.* Geneva: Aga Khan Foundation/World Health Organization.

Gillies, A. C. (1990) The quality of images as a measurement of image processing operator performance in fringe analysis. *Journal of Photographic Science*, **38**, 135–9 (based on a paper presented at the Royal Photographic Society Symposium on the Quantification of Images, Cambridge, 1989).

Gillies, A. C. (1996) *Software Quality*, 2nd edn. London: Chapman & Hall.

CHAPTER 4

Process Improvement

4.1   CHAPTER SUMMARY

This chapter considers how the ideas of process improvement have developed over the last fifty years. We shall consider the origins of the techniques in manufacturing before discussing how the techniques have spread first to other commercial sectors, then to the public sector. This will allow us to evaluate how useful these techniques are in the healthcare sector.

The next section focuses upon current methods in total quality management, or continuous quality improvement (CQI) as it is usually known in healthcare. The intension is to show that the techniques developed in other areas are in fact the basis for CQI and clinical audit in healthcare.

The final section examines the ISO9000 series, an international standard for quality management systems. The text describes the elements of the standard, and discusses its impact upon the improvement of patient care.

4.2   CLASSICAL PROCESS IMPROVEMENT

The area of process improvement is dominated by the ideas of a few key individuals who have become known as 'gurus'. Their words are given an almost religious significance by their 'disciples'. The most important of these 'gurus' are Deming, Juran and Crosby.

However, the origins of the technique go back to the First World

War when the quality of ammunition supplied to the troops was very poor. Testing was very limited, and so statistical and inspection techniques were developed to prevent errors earlier in the production chain by trying to detect faulty shells.

There is a certain irony in the parallels between the munitions production techniques of the 1914–18 war and the current emphasis upon preventing illness rather than curing it once it has occurred.

The man generally credited with inventing 'process improvement' in its modern form is Dr Edward Deming. However, Deming's basic principle was the same: instead of producing faulty items, improve the process to prevent errors occurring in the first place. Following the Second World War, he offered his ideas on quality to US government and industrial leaders. The ideas were not well received at the time. This error has ensured immortality for Dr Deming in the light of subsequent events. Deming was posted to Japan to help with the census there. He contacted the JUSU (The Union of Japanese Scientists and Engineers) about his ideas. Together with the ideas of Juran on fitness for purpose, the ideas of Deming formed the basis for Japanese economic recovery and subsequent Japanese domination of the world market. In time, his own country welcomed him back with the guilt of those who know they were wrong and have made a costly mistake.

Once the proof of Deming's and Juran's ideas was seen in the successful recovery of Japanese manufacturing industry, their ideas were rapidly accepted, particularly back home in the United States, where they were joined as quality 'gurus' by Phil Crosby, the man famous for 'zero defects' and a book entitled *Quality is Free*. This dominance by a few personalities, and particularly the often uncritical acceptance of their ideas, has not been universally well received.

There is a backlash currently being witnessed in some quarters. Total quality management (TQM) and its variants including continuous quality improvement (CQI) are currently very fashionable, and this inevitably leads to a scepticism amongst those who have seen other fashions come and go. Many articles on the subject reinforce the view that the 'gurus' are treated with uncritical respect.

In a culture such as the healthcare sector where there is already scepticism about the role of management, the attempt to introduce any new management technique is likely to be treated with suspicion.

The history of the subject of process improvement is largely the development of the ideas of Deming, Juran and Crosby. They each have different emphases and offer varying, if complementary, approaches to process improvement.

Dr Edward Deming's background is in statistics. His definition of quality is:

> A predictable degree of uniformity and dependability at low cost and suited to the market (Deming, 1986).

This definition is closely aligned with Garvin's manufacturing view of quality, which is unsurprising in view of the historical background to his ideas. However, his background in statistics leads to a strong advocacy of statistical quality control. He also strongly favours employee participation in decision making. He argues that it is insufficient for employees to do their best, that they must know what to do. For this reason he is opposed to the poster campaigns promoting quality found in many organizations, arguing they are misdirected and can cause frustration and resentment. He suggests 14 points for management, which should be used both internally and by suppliers:

- Constancy of purpose.
- A new philosophy.
- Cease dependence on inspection.
- End lowest tender contracts.
- Improve every process.
- Institute training on the job.
- Institute leadership.
- Drive out fear.
- Break down barriers.
- Eliminate exhortations.
- Eliminate targets.
- Permit pride of workmanship.
- Encourage education.
- Create top management structures.

Deming is a believer in single-sourcing of supplies, arguing that the benefits of a strong cooperative relationship with suppliers more than outweighs the short-term cost gains from competitive tendering. He advocates complete cooperation with suppliers, including the use of statistical process control (SPC) techniques, described below, to ensure the quality of incoming supplies.

Juran rose to fame with Deming in postwar Japan. He is credited with coining the phrase 'fitness for purpose', and is therefore particularly influential when we come to consider the use of process improvement ideas in software development. He has argued strongly that definitions of quality based upon 'conformance to specification' are inadequate. His approach is not dissimilar to that of Deming, and where it differs it is often complementary. This is not always true when we compare the ideas of Juran with those of Crosby. For example, Deming and Juran both argue against poster campaigns exhorting staff to achieve perfection. They both favour the use of SPC techniques, although Juran counsels against a 'tool-based approach'. However, Juran rejects both the main thrusts of Crosby's approach, 'zero defects' and 'conformance to specification'. He argues further that the law of diminishing returns applies to quality control and that 'quality is NOT free'. Juran has produced ten steps to quality improvement:

- Build awareness of need and opportunity for improvement.
- Set goals for improvement.
- Organize to reach the goals.
- Provide training.
- Carry out projects to solve problems.
- Report progress.
- Give recognition.
- Communicate results.
- Keep score.
- Maintain momentum by making annual improvement part of the regular process of the company.

Juran's approach is very much people-oriented. Thus, it places a strong emphasis upon teamwork and a project-based approach.

The third principal guru is Crosby. His approach, as has already been suggested, diverges from that of the other two gurus, especially Juran. He is best known for originating the concept of 'zero defects' and for the provocative title of one of his books, *Quality is Free* (Crosby, 1986). His approach may be summarized as prevention, rather than the traditional inspection and testing procedures. He equates prevention with perfection and this is often the prevalent view expressed today, particularly in the manufacturing arena, where Crosby's ideas seem most appropriate. He suggests a three-point 'quality vaccine'. This is intended to prevent non-conformance, the *bête noire* of the Crosby approach. The vaccine consists of determination, education and implementation. He proposes four 'absolutes' of quality:

- *definition*: conformance to requirements
- *system*: prevention
- *performance standard*: zero defects
- *measurement*: the price of non-conformance.

He too offers 14 steps to improvement, targeted at management:

- Make it clear that management is committed to quality.
- Form quality improvement teams with each department represented.
- Determine where current and potential problems lie.
- Evaluate the cost of quality and explain its use as a tool.
- Raise the quality awareness and concern of all employees.
- Take actions to correct problems identified.
- Establish a committee for the 'zero defects' programme.
- Train supervisors to actively carry out their role in quality improvement.
- Hold a 'zero defects day' for all employees to highlight the changes.
- Encourage individuals to establish improvement goals.
- Encourage communication with management about obstacles to improvement.
- Recognize and appreciate participants.
- Establish quality councils to aid communication.
- Do it all over again to show it never ends.

Whilst the results obtained in applying these ideas in manufacturing have been impressive, more doubts must be expressed about their applicability in a healthcare setting. In particular, the ideas of Crosby are particularly manufacturing-oriented and therefore least appropriate for healthcare for the following reasons:

(a) The approach is process, not people, oriented.

(b) It emphasizes conformance to specification and this view of quality is of limited use in healthcare.
(c) It is difficult to accept that there are absolutes in quality in any domain: if there are, then they are likely to be more subtle than the four pillars of Crosby's case.

The three principal approaches are compared below in Table 4.1.

From the historical origins of process improvement have come a number of techniques. The principal techniques are quality management, quality assurance and quality improvement. Quality management requires both quality assurance and improvement:

- *Quality assurance* is concerned with the systematic testing of services to ensure that quality is being delivered.
- *Quality improvement* is concerned with the improvement of quality through improvements in the process under scrutiny.

Deming saw quality assurance as a necessary step to improvement. However, as we shall see later, in healthcare and other sectors, quality assurance is often the dominant activity.

4.3   TECHNIQUES FOR CONTINUOUS QUALITY IMPROVEMENT

Quality management is achieved through the implementation of a quality management system (QMS). In ISO8042, the International Standards Organisation defined a quality management system as:

> The organisational structure, responsibilities, procedures, processes and resources for implementing quality management. (ISO, 1986)

The QMS provides a structure to ensure that the process is carried out in a formal and systematic way. Within software development, the adoption of a structured methodology may often provide the basis for a QMS. However, the QMS goes further than a methodology in ensuring that responsibility is clearly established for the prescribed procedures and processes. If the methodology is intended to lay down which procedures should be

Table 4.1 Comparison of principal ideas (after Oakland, 1989)

	Crosby	*Deming*	*Juran*
Definition	Conformance to requirements	Predictable degree of uniformity and dependability at low cost	Fitness for purpose
Senior management responsibility	Responsible for quality	Responsible for 94% of problems	Responsible for > 80% of problems
Performance standard	Zero defects	Many scales: use SPC, NOT zero defects	Avoid campaigns to exhort perfection
General approach	Prevention	Reduce variability: continuous improvement	Emphasis on management of human aspects
Structure	14 steps	14 points	10 steps
SPC	Rejects statistically acceptable level of quality	SPC must be used	Recommends SPC, but cautions against tool-based approach

Basis for improvement	A process, not a programme	Continuous: eliminate goals	Project based approach: set goals
Teamwork	Quality improvement teams: quality councils	Employee participation in decisions	Team/quality circle approach
Costs of quality	Quality is free!	No optimum, continuous improvement	Optimum, quality is NOT free
Purchasing	Supplier is extension of business	Use SPC through strong cooperation	Complex problems, use formal surveys
Vendor rating	Yes	No	Yes, but work with suppliers
Single sourcing of supply	Yes	Yes	No

carried out, the QMS should ensure that the procedures are actually carried out to the required standard.

At best, the QMS provides a disciplined and systematic framework. At worst, it can become a bureaucratic nightmare. Some people experiencing this scenario have dismissed the QMS as a system for 'the better documentation of errors'. This misses out on a vital part of any QMS, the requirement for continual improvement to correct the errors documented.

Thus, an essential part of any QMS is a feedback loop, possibly first suggested by Shewhart, but made famous by Deming as the 'plan–do–check–act' wheel (Fig. 4.1). The influence of this cycle cannot be overestimated. It is the basis for nearly all process improvement activity and is the basis of the methods used in healthcare known as continuous quality improvement (CQI) and clinical audit.

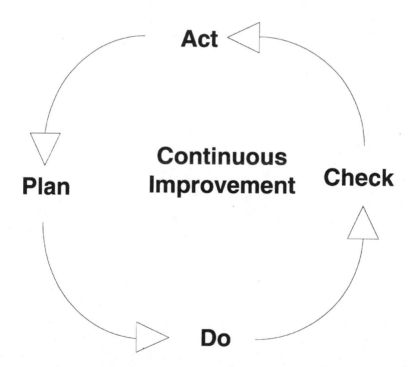

Figure 4.1 The plan–do–check–act wheel (after Deming, 1986, by permission of MIT and the W. Edwards Deming Institute. Published by MIT, copyright 1986 by the W. Edwards Deming Institute)

Total Quality Management

Quality management systems form the basis of total quality management (TQM). TQM is described by Oakland (1989) as:

> A method for ridding people's lives of wasted effort by involving everybody in the process of improving the effectiveness of work, so that results are achieved in less time.

Kanji (1990) describes it thus:

> Quality is to satisfy customer's requirements continually. Total quality is to achieve quality at low cost. Total quality management is to obtain total quality by involving everyone's daily commitment.

The term is rapidly becoming *passé*. However, the techniques underpinning it remain the basis of modern quality management methods.

We shall use one of the modern variants in terminology, continuous quality improvement (CQI), because it is favoured in healthcare and emphasizes the need for improvement as well as monitoring current practice. TQM is often misunderstood, perhaps because of the publicity that Crosby's 'zero defects' idea has attracted. In the mind of the author, total quality management refers to the involvement of all people and all processes within the quality management exercise. It does not imply, promise or guarantee perfection. One of the lessons from the experience of other sectors with these techniques is that they do not work unless they involve management and professionals. The culture found in many healthcare systems where there is a division between management and professionals is not conducive to success.

Neither is the blind introduction of commercial and business practices into the healthcare sector. The Japanese manufacturers who pioneered these techniques pursued them not out of any interest in quality itself but rather because they believed that it would increase profitability in the long run. This is the case for healthcare. Any application of ideas requires a sensitivity towards the needs of the sector.

Many clinical staff have been demotivated by listening to

'experts' from large commercial concerns ostensibly talking about quality programmes, but actually extolling the virtues of their organization. In particular such speakers never refer in public to the problems they experienced along the way in case they detract from the image of their company. These would provide some of the most useful lessons.

Rather than embark on a description of CQI, this chapter will consider the statistical and human management aspects of the technique, both crucial to successful implementation.

Statistical Process Control

Statistics are used to monitor performance as a first step to improvement. They are applied to a specific process, hence the name of the technique: statistical process control (SPC).

In order to monitor a process, it is necessary to define its inputs and outputs. The nature of the process is the operation of transforming the inputs into the outputs. The scope of the process must be clearly defined to prevent ambiguity.

SPC methods allow us to calculate levels of non-conformity and also provide a strategy for the reduction of variability. Many SPC techniques are very simple. Ishikawa (1985) has suggested seven basic tools for collection and analysis of quality data (Table 4.2).

Process flow charting is a diagramming technique to illustrate

Table 4.2   SPC techniques

SPC technique	Purpose
Process flow charting	To show what is done
Tally charts	To show how often it is done
Histograms	To show overall variations
Pareto analysis	To highlight big problems
Cause and effect (Ishikawa) diagrams	To indicate causes
Scatter diagrams	To highlight relationships
Control charts	To show which variations to control

the inputs and flow of a process. This technique is described in detail in Chapter 5 of Oakland (1989). An example is shown in Fig. 4.2.

Tally charts are used in conjunction with histograms to collect and display data. Tally chart forms should be clear and easy to use. Pareto analysis is designed to show what percentage of faults may be attributed to each cause. An example is shown in Fig. 4.3.

Cause and effect analysis is represented by an Ishikawa or fishbone diagram which maps the inputs affecting a quality problem (Fig. 4.4). The strength and orientation of correlations may be seen on scatter diagrams (Fig. 4.5). If the correlation is strong the points will be grouped around a line of best fit. The gradient of this line may be found by regression analysis. A positive gradient indicates a positive correlation, a negative gradient indicates a negative correlation.

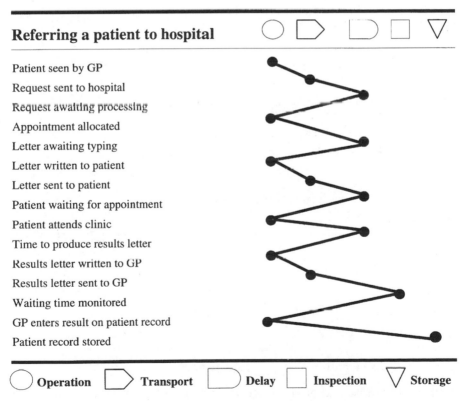

Figure 4.2   A sample process flow diagram

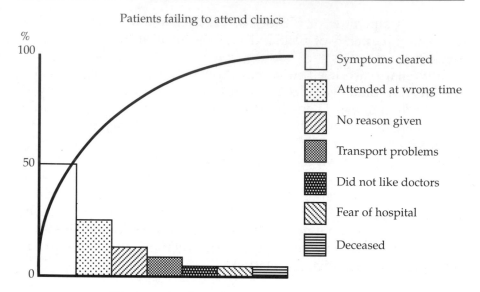

Figure 4.3   Sample Pareto analysis graph

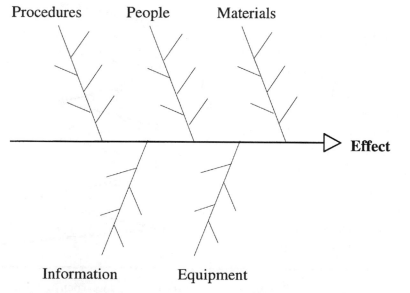

Figure 4.4   Cause and effect diagrams (after Ishikawa, 1985, reproduced by permission of Prentice Hall)

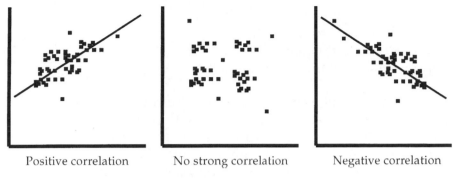

| Positive correlation | No strong correlation | Negative correlation |

Figure 4.5 Scatter plots

Control charts are used to monitor how a parameter (e.g. the number of defectors) varies over time through the process. Other more sophisticated techniques such as regression analysis may be employed but the additional effort required is rarely repaid in terms of a better understanding of the data.

Like many TQM ideas, SPC methods were first developed in the manufacturing area. They require some adaptation to healthcare if they are to be put to good use. A discussion of some of the issues arising from the use of SPC techniques in 'non-product' applications is given by Bissell (1990).

Human Factors: Establishing a Quality Culture

There are two important parts to a QMS. There are the tools and procedures, discussed above, and then there are the people. All the procedures, tools and techniques are only there to enable the people to achieve a quality result.

Staff acceptance is therefore vital. This will not happen by itself. The management of change is critical to the success of the process. The system can only work if staff perceive the benefits to themselves. These include the potential for:

- greater job satisfaction
- less time spent on pointless activity
- less money wasted

- greater pride in work
- better treatment for patients
- more group participation
- more staff input into the way they do their job.

These benefits will accrue only in a culture where managers and clinicians work together. Oakland (1989) points out that staff will not be well motivated towards a quality programme in the absence of top management commitment and action, an organizational quality climate and a team approach to quality problems. It is particularly important that communication be a two-way process. For staff to be motivated, they must feel 'involved' and that their contribution and ideas will make a difference. Further they must see that cost savings result in better treatment for their patients.

One of the principal means suggested for getting staff involved is through the use of quality circles. A quality circle is a group of workers who are asked, not told, to join. They will generally have a trained leader, who might be their foreman or line manager. There should be an overall supervisor to coordinate the whole quality circle programme throughout an organization. Finally, management must be committed to the programme. Whilst they retain the right and obligation to manage, they must not reject recommendations without good reason or they will strangle the idea at birth.

Quality circles are generally made up of between three and fifteen people. Larger than this and the group becomes fragmented, with some members opting out. The author strongly recommends a group size in single figures to obtain maximum benefit. Meetings are better if held at a site away from the work area. Optimum frequency of meetings appears to vary from one to three weeks, depending upon the problems under consideration.

The circle should decide for itself which problem to consider, although management usually retains the right of a polite veto. The circle may call in outside experts in the role of consultants, but the decision making and problem solving role must remain within the circle. Quality circles will not simply happen. Training is a vital ingredient in the success of a quality circle. The leader needs to be trained in encouraging people to contribute, in structuring a discussion and ensuring that the group is not dominated by one or two characters. The team members need training in basic quality techniques so that they know how problems may be solved.

An alternative, but complementary, approach to organizing for quality is the quality improvement team (QIT), an idea apparently originating with Crosby, to tackle a specific problem. It brings together a blend of knowledge, skills and experience in a multi-disciplinary approach. The optimum size of a QIT is typically five to ten people. The life of a QIT is likely to be limited, as they come into being to address a specific problem. It is important to create a stimulating environment for discussion and to encourage people to think creatively. It is likely that obvious solutions have already been tried and discarded before the QIT comes into being. It is therefore probable that a genuine solution will arise from a piece of 'lateral thinking'. Each member has been invited to join the team because of their expertise. What appears to be a fanciful thought may in fact be the start of a solution.

In a recent discussion on problem solving strategies, in which the author was involved, it was pointed out that many tricky problems were difficult to solve because to reach the solution or goal state, it was necessary to take a first step in what was apparently the wrong direction. This can make team leadership very tricky. The division between 'lateral thinking' and irrelevance can be difficult to spot. It can also prove difficult to build up a team identity when its existence is ephemeral and success will inevitably lead to the group disbanding.

As with other techniques, QITs are offered as another tool. On their own, they will not cause a revolution but they can make a useful contribution to an overall programme. They should be seen as complementary to quality circles rather than conflicting.

Table 4.3 compares the two techniques discussed above.

Juran is a strong advocate of team working practices as a way of motivating people towards quality. The advantages cited by Oakland (1989) for team working include:

- a greater variety of problems may be tackled
- a greater variety of skills, knowledge and expertise is available
- the approach is more satisfying and builds team morale
- cross-departmental problems can be dealt with more easily
- recommendations carry more weight.

Table 4.3 A comparative summary of quality circles and quality improvement teams

	Quality improvement team	Quality circle
Purpose	To bring together specific expertise to solve a particular problem	To allow workers the chance to contribute ideas to solve problems occurring
Membership	Five to ten experts from a range of disciplines	Up to fifteen 'front line' workers
Led by	Person most concerned with task success	Foreman/line manager
Lifetime	Limited	Ongoing
Training needs	Need to work as group	Basic quality methods

The author agrees with all these comments but notes some cautions from observing team working in action, especially in the healthcare sector. There are many divisions to be overcome between clinician and manager, doctor and nurse, between different clinical specialties, between primary and secondary care and so on. Where team working is clearly advantageous, some progress has been made. However, in areas such as process improvement, the participants are likely to be unconvinced of the benefits and this may therefore not provide enough incentive to tackle cultural barriers.

The teams need to work internally in close proximity. Personality clashes can be exaggerated within a confined group. This may be addressed by the use of personality profiling. Some people say this can help to assemble compatible groups, others disagree. Some people find adapting to the new way of working very difficult and may be more isolated as a consequence. Tensions can arise between different groups because of different priorities.

One of the biggest problems that can arise in any organization, whether team-based or not, is a lack of appreciation of the interdependence of each contribution. A hospital is a complex organization and each functional group is dependent upon others. This leads to the concept of 'internal' and 'external' customers. An internal customer is anyone who receives a service or product from another group or individual. There is a growing perception of the value of the concept of the 'internal' customer, sometimes referred to in terms of a 'quality chain'.

The use of the term 'customer' may be disliked in terms of healthcare. However, the analysis of customers as internal and external and the recognition that the patient is only one of many customers is important.

Consider a patient attending a hospital for an outpatient appointment at an orthopaedic clinic. The external customers of the clinic are the patient, their family doctor, and ultimately the government and the taxpayer as the funding provider. The clinic is in turn an internal customer of the support services of the hospital including, but not limited to, patient admissions, X-ray, cleaning, technical support. The quality chain is illustrated in Fig. 4.6. The clinic, as an internal customer of the support services, depends upon the quality of service provided in order to provide a good quality of care to the patient and meet the needs of the other external customers. In this sense a 'quality chain' exists which means the quality of care depends upon each link in that chain.

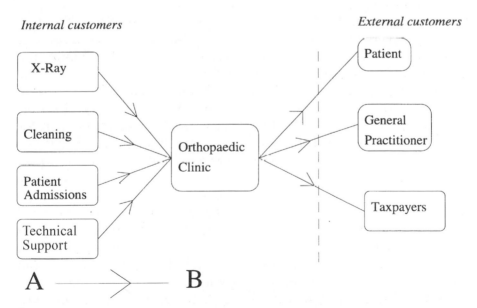

Figure 4.6 Customer analysis of an orthopaedic clinic (B is a customer of A)

In managing any situation, a large factor in the success is not connected with the procedures employed, but with the day-to-day running of the organization. It has been one of the criticisms of TQM in other sectors that it focuses upon procedures and that procedures can help and facilitate or indeed they can obstruct and hinder. What they cannot do is to guarantee success. This must ultimately depend upon the performance of the people concerned, who may choose to take advantage of the help provided by systems or procedures or not. The problem in trying to analyse the factors at work is that they are often difficult to generalize and are strongly influenced by personalities and specific environments. We shall, therefore, consider first the environment and then take two stereotypical personality types which form the extremes of a spectrum.

Top-down or Bottom-up?

A tension exists in any organization where a quality culture is being established. The tension exists between a force acting from the top down and a force coming up from the bottom. The top-down force is the 'desire to manage'. Management is absolutely necessary. It is not possible to achieve quality by committee. Without firm management, there will be no policy, no strategy, no consistency in decision making, and chaos will ensue.

However, there is a clear need to feed ideas up the organization. A quality culture will actually increase the flow of ideas from the workforce. Strong management can verge on autocracy. What one person might regard as a well organized stable environment may in fact be stagnant rather than stable. People with ideas which conflict with those of management can be seen as troublemakers. A perception that the last person to have an idea was sacked for it will not encourage others to come forward. There are no clear rules on this. Ask a well-regarded manager the principles he or she uses and you may well be quoted a set of ideas and statements. Ask how he or she does the job and the manager will probably use phrases such as 'by experience' or 'one instinctively knows'. Intuition ultimately plays a large part in managing people. This is unhelpful when trying to identify best practice. It is even less helpful when a badly regarded manager says the same thing!

Most work on quality management assumes that the starting point is a hierarchical management structure and the need is to flatten this structure. However, healthcare organizational structures are more complex, involving management and clinical hierarchies. As well as flattening each hierarchy there is a need for integration of structures.

A balance between structure, direction and policy on the one hand and innovation, lateral thinking and creativity on the other is required. Views of quality which emphasize conformance in components can too easily lead to an emphasis on conformance when dealing with staff. There is a time for doing things 'by the book' and a time for not. One of the best definitions of an expert is someone who knows when the rule book can be safely discounted.

Managing People: the Stereotypes

The First Stereotype: the Cynic

The cynic has been there, seen it, done it and heard it all before. He or she appears to have been at Deming's inaugural lecture in Japan and knows that it won't work. This sort of person can be very destructive in many situations. However, they can also offer much:

- They are usually experienced staff with a wealth of experiential knowledge which could be usefully exploited.
- The role of devil's advocate can be an extremely useful one, particularly in the situation where outside consultants have been employed.
- They are likely to become strong advocates of good practice if they can be convinced. How often have you heard, 'Well, of course, I always thought ...' shortly after a U-turn of amazing proportions?

One strategy is to try to carve out a role for such a person which exploits their strengths of experience and scepticism whilst trying to insulate many other younger impressionable staff from their negative attitude. Many cynics will thrive on being given such a role.

The Second Stereotype: the Enthusiast

Enthusiasm is a valuable commodity but it can cause as many headaches as it solves. Enthusiasm tends to be short-lived. People who become enthusiastic tend to get bored and move on to the next idea that comes along. Enthusiasm can also lead people to be uncritical and not to see potential pitfalls until it is too late. It might seem an attractive proposition to put our enthusiast and cynic together, as the best of both would be almost ideal. However, such a combination is likely to be destructive before it ever bears fruit. Rather than put the two together it is often more useful to allow their influences on a group of people to balance each other out. If this can be achieved without bringing the two bodies together in an explosive combination, then the net effect may be beneficial.

The role of the enthusiast should be to feed other people with ideas and enthusiasm. The group being fed will filter out the more zany ideas at the start. However, it is hoped they will adopt and develop some of the ideas at least. These embryonic ideas may then be exposed to the sceptical gaze of our cynic, under which more will wither and perish. The ideas remaining are likely to be both useful and sustaining. It is rare though very valuable to find a creative enthusiast with the potential to develop their ideas.

Fortunately, perhaps, most people fall between our two stereotypical images. However, the balance between nurturing creativity and maintaining structure can be tricky. Ensuring that everyone has a role to play in a workforce aiming at quality is a challenge and reinforces the views of all three gurus, that ultimately the buck stops with senior management.

4.4 THE ISO9001 STANDARD

Standards are generally defined in terms of a model of best practice, against which all others may be compared. This is true of the standards available for quality management systems.

The ISO9000 series of standards (also known as BS5750 and EN29000) are widely applied to quality management systems in many different disciplines. The standards establish a model of a QMS to be employed, and then the certification body (e.g. BSI QA in the UK for the ISO9000 series) is called in to ensure that the implementation meets the required standard and indeed continues to meet the required standard over time.

It is vital to understand that a standard neither improves quality directly, nor ensures perfection. It should, however, ensure that the correct procedures are in place and being carried out. The standard provides a model, and the certification procedure the incentive to ensure that things are done correctly.

Promoters of the standards argue that because they are generic management standards they may be employed in both commercial and non-commercial organizations across a wide range of products and services. We shall scrutinize this claim in the context of healthcare later in this section.

There are range of standards defined according to the scope of activity undertaken by the organization (Table 4.4). The series dates from 1979, when BS5750 was introduced in the UK. In 1987, the corresponding ISO, BS and EN standards were harmonized to

Table 4.4   The ISO9000 series of quality management standards

ISO	*EN*	*BS*	*Description*
ISO9000	EN29000	BS5750 pt0	A guide to selecting the appropriate standard for a quality management system
ISO9001	EN29001	BS5750 pt1	The specification of a QMS for design, development, production, installation and service
ISO9002	EN29002	BS5750 pt2	The specification of a QMS for production and installation
ISO9003	EN29003	BS5750 pt3	The specification of a QMS for final inspection and testing
ISO9004	EN29004	BS5750 pt4	Guidance in setting up a QMS to meet the ISO9001/2/3 standards

produce three identical series of standards. In this text, we shall use the ISO numbers for consistency. The three main standards are ISO9001, 9002 and 9003. ISO9001 is intended for applications where there is a significant design element. ISO9002 is intended for many manufacturing situations where the product is produced to a predefined specification, and ISO9003 for simple applications where the quality can be determined by a simple final inspection and testing procedure. ISO9000 provides guidance on which standard to adopt, and ISO9004 assistance on how to establish a QMS which meets the requirements of the ISO9000 series.

In this section, we shall deal with the requirements of the ISO9001 standard. The ISO9002 and ISO9003 standards may be thought of as subsets of the ISO9001 standard. The standard is based on a model specification for a quality management system, adopting two fundamental principles:

- right first time
- fitness for purpose.

The standard is intended to be realistic and implementable and, therefore, sets no prescriptive quality performance targets, referring instead to standards agreed as part of the contract with the customer and acceptable to them. The standard focuses upon ensuring that procedures are carried out in a systematic way and that the results are documented, again in a systematic manner.

The main requirements are dealt with in Clause 4 of the standard under 20 subclauses: the headings are summarized in Table 4.5. Those clauses also found in ISO9002 and ISO9003 are shown in the right-hand columns. It should be noted that in ISO 9003, some of the clauses are simplified.

Clause 4.1: Management Responsibility

The model recognizes the importance of management responsibility for quality throughout the organization. Whilst it is impossible for senior management to personally oversee everything, the standard explicitly provides for a management representative who is directly responsible for quality and is accountable to senior management.

This clause also sets out the basic principles for establishing the

Table 4.5 Requirements of the ISO9000 standards

Clause	ISO9001	ISO9002	ISO9003
4.1	Management responsibility	Yes	Yes
4.2	Quality system	Yes	Yes
4.3	Contract review	Yes	
4.4	Design control		
4.5	Document control	Yes	Yes
4.6	Purchasing	Yes	
4.7	Purchaser supplied product	Yes	
4.8	Product identification and traceability	Yes	Yes
4.9	Process control	Yes	
4.10	Inspection and testing	Yes	Yes
4.11	Inspection, measuring and testing equipment	Yes	Yes
4.12	Inspection and testing status	Yes	Yes
4.13	Control of non-conforming product	Yes	Yes
4.14	Corrective action	Yes	
4.15	Handling, storage, packaging and delivery	Yes	Yes
4.16	Quality records	Yes	Yes
4.17	Internal quality audits	Yes	
4.18	Training	Yes	Yes
4.19	Servicing		
4.20	Statistical techniques	Yes	Yes

quality system within the organization and sets out many of its functions, which are then described in greater detail in later sections.

Clause 4.2: Quality System

The model requires the organization to set up a quality system. The system should be documented and a quality plan and manual prepared. The scope of the plan is determined by the activities undertaken and consequently the standard (ISO9001/2/3) employed. The focus of the plan should be to ensure that activities are carried out in a systematic way and documented.

Clause 4.3: Contract Review

Contract review specifies that each customer order should be regarded as a contract. Order entry procedures should be developed and documented. The aim of these procedures is to:

- ensure that customer requirements are clearly defined in writing
- highlight differences between the order and the original quotation, so that they may be agreed
- ensure that the requirements can be met.

The aim of this clause is to ensure that both the supplier and customer understand the specified requirements of each order and to document this agreed specification to prevent misunderstandings and conflict at a later date.

Clause 4.4: Design Control

Design control procedures are required to control and verify design activities, to take the results from market research through to practical designs. The key activities covered are:

- planning for research and development
- assignment of activities to qualified staff
- identification of interfaces between relevant groups
- preparation of a design brief
- production of technical data
- verification that the output from the design phase meets the input requirements
- identification and documentation of all changes and modifications.

The aim of this section is to ensure that the design phase is carried out effectively and to ensure that the output from the design phase accurately reflects the input requirements.

Clause 4.5: Document Control

Three levels of documentation are recognized by the standard:

- Level 1: planning and policy documents
- Level 2: procedures
- Level 3: detailed instructions.

The top level documents the quality plan and sets out policy on key quality issues. Each level adds more detail to the documentation. Where possible existing documentation should be incorporated. The aim should be to provide systematic documentation, rather than simply to provide more documents. It is important that each level of documentation be consistent with the one above it, providing greater detail as each level is descended.

It is a common complaint that the standard requires a prohibitive amount of documentation to be produced. Supporters of the standard argue that systemizing of documentation can actually lead to a reduction in volume owing to the removal of obsolete and surplus documents. It is more likely that some reduction will be achieved, which will offset greater volumes in other areas.

Good existing documentation should be incorporated into any new system and this is facilitated by the standard not specifying a particular format, but merely specifying that documents be fit for their intended purpose.

Clause 4.6: Purchasing

The purchasing system is designed to ensure that all purchased products and services conform to the requirements and standards of the organization. The emphasis should be placed upon verifying the supplier's own quality management procedures. Where a supplier has also obtained external certification for their quality management systems, checks may be considerably simplified. As with all procedures, they should be documented.

Clause 4.7: Purchaser Supplied Product

All services and products supplied by the customer must be checked for suitability, in the same way as supplies purchased from any other supplier. In order to ensure this, procedures should be put in place and documented, so that these services and products may be traced through all processes and storage.

Clause 4.8: Product Identification and Traceability

To ensure effective process control and to correct any non-conformance, it is necessary to establish procedures to identify and trace materials from input to output. This also enables quality problems to be traced to root causes. It may be that the problem may be traced back to supplied materials, in which case the problem may lie outside the quality system altogether.

Clause 4.9: Process Control

Process control requires a detailed knowledge of the process itself. This must be documented, often in graphical form, as a process flow chart or similar. Procedures for setting up or calibration must also be recorded. Documented instructions should be available to staff to ensure that they have the capability to carry out the task as specified.

It is staggering how often organizations do not understand their own processes properly. The discipline of documenting the actual process precisely and unambiguously for certification purposes can be very educational.

Clause 4.10: Inspection and Testing

Inspection and testing are required to ensure conformance in three stages:

- incoming materials or services
- in process
- finished product and/or service.

All incoming supplies must be checked in some way. The method will vary according to the status of the supplier's quality management procedures, from full examination to checking evidence supplied with the goods.

Monitoring 'in process' is required to ensure all is going according to plan. At the end of the process, any final inspection tests documented in the quality plan must be carried out. Evidence of conformity to quality standards together with details of any supporting 'in-process' monitoring may be included. In an effective system, however, the final inspection and test should not have to be as extensive as it otherwise would be. In addition, it should not reveal many problems, since they should have been eliminated by this stage.

Clause 4.11: Inspection, Measuring and Testing Equipment

Any equipment used for measuring and testing must be calibrated and maintained. Procedures to ensure that calibration and maintenance activities are properly implemented should be documented, identifying the measurements required and the precision associated with each. Records must be kept of all activity.

Checking and calibration activities should become part of regular maintenance. Management should ensure that checks are carried out at the prescribed intervals and efficient records kept.

Clause 4.12: Inspection and Testing Status

All material and services may be classified in one of three categories:

- awaiting inspection or test
- passed inspection
- failed inspection.

This status should be clearly identifiable at any stage. It is important that material awaiting inspection is not mistakenly allowed to miss inspection at any stage as non-conformance may go undetected.

Clause 4.13: Control of Non-Conforming Product

The standard defines non-conforming product as all products or services falling outside tolerance limits agreed in advance with the customer. Once again it is not prescriptive about performance levels. All non-conforming products or services should be clearly identified, documented and, if possible, physically separated from the conforming product. Procedures should be established to handle non-conforming products by reworking, disposal, regrading or other acceptable documented courses of action.

There are circumstances where the standard permits the sale of non-conforming product provided that the customer is clearly aware of the circumstances and is generally offered a concession. Representatives of certification bodies suggest that this is an area where organizations often become lax after a while, relaxing procedures and allowing non-conforming product through.

Clause 4.14: Corrective Action

Corrective action is the key to continual improvement. Such action should be implemented via a systematic programme which provides guidance and defines the duties of all parties. Records should be kept of any action taken so that future audits can investigate its effectiveness.

Clause 4.15: Handling, Storage, Packaging and Delivery

Handling and associated activities must be designed to protect the quality built into the product. Sub-contractors employed for transportation should be subject to the same documented procedures as internal employees. The scope of this clause is determined by the contract with the customer. The clause covers all activities which are the contractual obligation of the supplier.

Clause 4.16: Quality Records

Quality records are vital to ensure that quality activities have actually been carried out. They form the basis for quality audits, both internal and external. They do not have to conform to a prescribed format, but must be fit for their intended purpose. As many will exist before the accredited system is implemented, the aim is to systemize and assimilate existing practice wherever possible, to reduce wasted effort in reproducing previous work in this area.

Clause 4.17: Internal Quality Audits

The quality system should be 'policed' from within the organization and not be dependent upon external inspection. Procedures should be established to set up regular internal audits as part of normal management procedure. The role of internal audits should be to identify problems early in order to minimize their impact and cost.

Clause 4.18: Training

Training activities should be implemented and documented. In particular, written procedures are required:

- to establish training needs
- to carry out training activity
- to record the training requirements and completed activities for each member of staff.

It is a requirement of the standard that at all stages, the staff required to carry out a particular function have the skills, knowledge and tools necessary to do a proper job. Training refers not just to formal courses but to informal knowledge sharing as well.

Clause 4.19: Servicing

Where servicing procedures are required, they should be documented and verified. The procedures should ensure that servicing is actually carried out and that sufficient resources are available. It is necessary to set up good interfaces with the customer if this function is to be carried out effectively. The same monitoring procedures as are applied to internal processes should be carried out within the servicing function.

Clause 4.20: Statistical Techniques

Statistical techniques are required to be used where appropriate. The standard does not specify particular techniques or methods but does specify that once again they should be appropriate for the intended purpose. Their use may be necessary in order to satisfy other requirements, notably process control, detailed in Clause 4.9.

The Process of Seeking Certification

Organizations seeking a certification should first implement a quality system, in accordance with the requirements of the standard. This may require outside help, such as quality expertise provided by consultants. However, the most important requirement is gaining acceptance for the system internally at this stage. Once the system is accepted by the staff and has been operating for a few months to iron out inevitable teething troubles, then it is often advisable to have a pre-inspection quality audit carried out by a third party. This will highlight problems and if carried out effectively should ensure that the real inspection goes smoothly. Once this inspection has been carried out successfully, then the certification body should be contacted and the certification process proper started. They will require pre-inspection examination of the relevant documentation. They will then visit the organization to ensure that the system meets the required standard.

Once the conditions are satisfied, a certificate may be issued. This may be withdrawn at any time if the system is not properly maintained. Surprise inspection visits may be made twice a year after certification to ensure continuing conformance.

The ISO9001 Standard in Healthcare

ISO9001 has proved to be an extremely powerful incentive to organizations to get their quality procedures right. Further, certification is external evidence of this fact. However, there are arguments for its usefulness being limited within the healthcare area.

In spite of claims that the ISO9000 series is a universal and generic set of standards for quality management systems, it shows a strong bias towards commercial manufacturing. It strongly emphasizes quality assurance aspects and makes little attempt to facilitate quality improvement.

There is very little in the standard about establishing a human quality culture. It may be argued that such a culture is implicit within the model, and that it is necessary to meet the other requirements. The human element is too important to be left as an implicit requirement: its omission leaves the standard open to the accusation made by some that it is simply a record-keeping system. Without the establishment of a quality culture and a formal requirement for procedures to facilitate the process, the vital process of continuous improvement which takes quality management beyond the recording of errors and performance may be omitted.

It is worth examining where ISO9000 has been enthusiastically adopted. It is generally used as a marketing tool by commercial companies to demonstrate a basic level of quality procedures to their customers. It is not perceived primarily as a tool for improving quality but rather for improving the marketability of goods and services.

This may be demonstrated by the areas seeking and gaining ISO9000 certification within the UK National Health Service. With increasing commercialization, technical services are required to compete for contracts with external commercial organizations. In response to this, several departments have established quality management systems and gained ISO9000 certification.

This has enabled them to compete successfully with external firms for internal and external contracts. If this improves the quality of service provided then this will, through the quality chain, result in better care for the patient.

However, ISO9000 is not the dominant quality improvement mechanism in the NHS that it is becoming in many other sectors.

4.5   REFERENCES

Bissell, A. F. (1990) Multipositional process evaluation: an example and some general guidelines. *Total Quality Management*, **1**(1), 95–100.

Crosby, P. B. (1986) *Quality is Free*. Maidenhead: McGraw-Hill.

Deming, W. E. (1986) *Out of the Crisis*. Cambridge, MA: MIT Center for Advanced Engineering.

International Standards Organisation (1986) *ISO 8042: Quality Vocabulary*. Geneva: ISO (available from BSI, London).

International Standards Organisation (1994) *ISO 9000 Series: Standards for Quality Management Systems.* Geneva: ISO (available from BSI, London).

Ishikawa, K. (1985) *What is Total Quality Control? – The Japanese Way.* Englewood Cliffs, NJ: Prentice Hall.

Kanji, G. K. (1990) Total quality management: the second industrial revolution. *Total Quality Management,* **1**(1): 3–12.

Oakland, J. (1989) *Total Quality Management.* London: Heinemann.

CHAPTER 5

Clinical Audit

5.1 CHAPTER SUMMARY

This chapter will look at clinical audit. It will describe the basics of the process and relate it back to its antecedents. It will look at the context in which audit has grown up, and the way that this has influenced its nature.

The chapter will consider the role of computers and how computers have facilitated the growth of audit. However, it will also indicate where computers have distorted the growth of the audit process.

Finally, it will look at the pros and cons of the audit process as a quality improvement mechanism in healthcare.

5.2 THE CLINICAL AUDIT CYCLE

Clinical audit was introduced in 1989 in the White Paper *Working for Patients* (DoH, 1989). Since then the scope has been extended to all healthcare professions. Audit has been recognized as an activity involving all healthcare workers, and hence the term has changed from medical audit to clinical audit.

The process of clinical audit is defined in the audit cycle (Fig. 5.1) which shows a remarkable similarity to classical process improvement techniques pioneered by Deming and Shewhart, and described in the previous chapter (see Fig. 4.1).

Audit is not new. Aside from its links to process improvement,

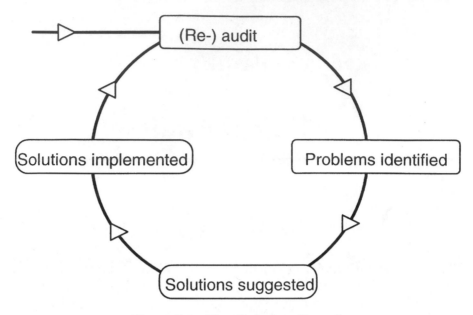

Figure 5.1   The clinical audit cycle

we can trace its roots back through the attempts of clinicians to improve their professional activities. For example:

- 1858: improved management of basic care: Florence Nightingale
- 1916: definition of standards and the need for confidentiality: Bowman and the US College of Surgeons
- 1952: voluntary collection of standard data on maternal mortality: UK Department of Health.

Clinical audits have a number of characteristics which most will share. They are locally organized and controlled. They are generally small-scale and have the stated aim of improving patient care. The latter is normally a condition of funding. Clinical audit is a 'bottom-up' approach to quality management.

Crucially, audits should result in changes in practice to effect change. They should be carried out in a systematic manner. They should be an ongoing process, or at the very least contain a commitment to re-audit to investigate the effect of changes.

The Department of Health definition from the 1989 White Paper sets out the desirable characteristics of the audit process. Audit should be:

- systematic
- analytical
- concerned with the quality of care.

This statement also outlines the scope of audit activity. It should cover:

- procedures for diagnosis and treatment
- the use of resources
- the resulting outcomes
- the impact upon the quality of life of the patient.

Audits are carried out by many different people with many different backgrounds. It is questionable whether the overall approach to clinical audit is indeed systematic and analytical. Individual audits show a wide variation in the techniques used and the scope considered.

Characteristics of Good Audit Practice

Within the Oxford region of the United Kingdom, the following characteristics are recommended for good audit practice (Hunt and Legg, 1992):

- appropriate design
- valid measures of quality of care
- reliable data
- peer review of findings
- problem identification
- effective action to eliminate or minimize problems
- evidence of improvement through re-audit.

Appropriate Design

Audits must be designed, not evolved. They are not a trawl for interesting data. They are not even a process designed to test a specific hypothesis. This is research. Audit is a systematic process intended to result in an improvement in patient care. Lessons for the effective design of audits are presented in Chapter 9.

Valid Measures of Quality of Care

Quality is notoriously difficult to measure as we have already seen. However, without measurement it is impossible to quantify current levels of performance and any subsequent improvement in patient care.

Reliable Data

The quality of data is a difficult one. Much audit activity is based upon non-verifiable case notes. The transcription process to enter these records into a computer is also error-prone. Gillies (1995) provides advice on good data handling practice. However, any audit is only as good as the data on which it is based.

Peer Review of Findings

Peer review is crucial to the implementation of change. Professional assessment is necessary to evaluate findings to distinguish the underlying causes of findings. Without the addition of professional judgement, statistics are meaningless.

Peer review will also help with identification of underlying causes, crucial to identification of effective change, and reduce resistance to change when implemented.

Problem Identification

Although purist process improvement authors such as Deming have argued that there is always room for improvement, audit effectively uses a sampling procedure to select areas to audit. The first criterion for problem selection, therefore, is that there should be a suspected problem.

Often, the problem will need to be refined. In order to carry out an appropriately focused audit, it is sensible to undertake a preliminary investigation to define the problem area more clearly.

Effective Action to Eliminate or Minimize Problems

In order to identify appropriate solutions, it will be necessary to identify underlying causes. This may not be obvious from the audit results. In spite of much effort to the contrary, many audits still fail to implement change. This is explored in the study in the next chapter.

Evidence of Improvement Through Re-audit

Even where change has been implemented, it is necessary to evaluate the effect of those changes through a re-audit.

5.3 VIEWS OF CLINICAL AUDIT

In spite of the Department of Health's definition there is diversity of practice in audit. To resolve these inconsistencies, we shall adopt again the approach of Garvin (1984) describing different 'views' of clinical audit (Fig. 5.2). This type of model is designed to provide a richer understanding by outlining alternative view-points, rather than seeking to establish one particular view as superior. In particular, in this section we shall propose an information management view.

The Process View

The process view is based upon classical process improvement ideas first proposed by Deming (1986) and Juran (1979) over forty years ago in the context of the Japanese manufacturing industry. Proponents of this view point to the similarity of the clinical audit cycle to the process improvement cycle as detailed in the previous section (see Figures 5.1 and 4.1).

Process improvement may be considered under two headings:

- measurement of existing performance
- improvement of performance.

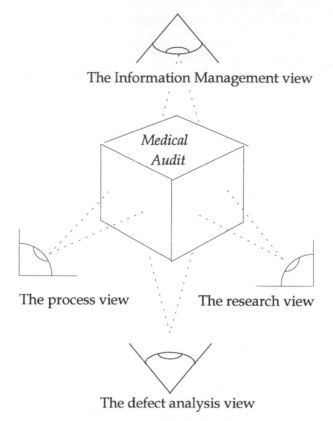

The Information Management view

Medical
Audit

The process view   The research view

The defect analysis view

Figure 5.2   Views of clinical audit

In quality terms, these activities are represented as quality assurance (QA) and quality improvement (QI).

Quality assurance in service organizations is generally monitored through quality audits, where the processes in place in an organization are evaluated to see whether they are being carried out consistently and effectively. In the same way, clinical audit may be regarded as monitoring the effectiveness of all the processes contributing to patient care. This view suggests that it is just as important to monitor processes such as communication with patients as it is to evaluate the clinical procedures they undergo.

One implication of the quality assurance view of clinical audit is that audit measures performance against a benchmark. However, to fully represent the process improvement cycle, clinical audit

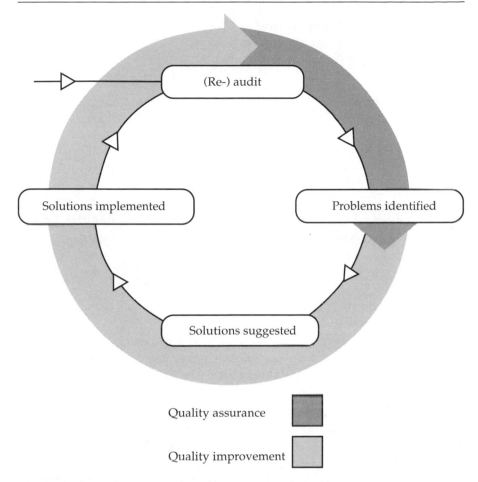

Figure 5.3   The quality assurance and improvement stages of the audit
cycle

must include quality improvement. It is not enough to measure
performance, but rather to use those measures to improve performance by feeding back the results of the audit study to highlight problem areas and facilitate process improvement (Fig. 5.3).

The process view is the closest to that enshrined in the foundation documents of clinical audit (DoH, 1989). However, because of
a number of barriers, it is not necessarily the dominant view in
practice. Those barriers include:

• organizational culture amongst clinicians

- data gathering and collection
- meaningful performance measurement
- ad hoc and fragmented practice.

The Research View

The view that people have depends upon their background. For example, many doctors coming from a research background draw comparisons with research. The importance of the research view in clinical audit is based upon the culture in which much audit activity takes place. It is an activity which many doctors feel is much more professionally respectable than quality assurance. It is a domain in which they are the leaders, rather than quality assurance where managers are often perceived to take the lead role.

However, there are some crucial differences between research and audit activity. Clinical audit borrows from research in a number of areas. It is clearly an investigation which may be based upon one or more hypotheses. These may be investigated according to classical scientific methods, in a similar manner to a clinical research project.

Consider as an example an audit carried out in the Oxford Region. This looked at the experience of surgeons carrying out a specific clinical procedure (laparoscopy and dye test). The audit was set up to investigate the quality of care associated with this procedure in an infertility clinic. Principally, the audit wished to address the question of the experience of the operators carrying out the procedure.

The procedure was a complex one and expert opinion suggested that it should be carried out only by consultants, because they had the greatest experience. However, the audit was based upon the assumption that this was not the case in the hospital in question. A hypothesis was therefore derived:

> Currently, laparoscopy and dye tests are carried out by a range of personnel.

The next stage was to test this hypothesis by looking at patient records. In this case a set of records was considered covering a 17-

month period, of those who had undergone a laparoscopy and dye test between the dates 1 January 1992 and 30 May 1993. The hypothesis was tested by considering the status of the surgeon in a total of 80 cases from four surgical teams, each led by a consultant. The hypothesis proved to be correct.

However, this link between the classical scientific research method and audit is only superficial and if taken at a deeper level can lead to misleading assumptions about the purpose of research and audit.

In particular, audit problems are generally well-defined and have clear aims and objectives. Research problems are generally fuzzier with less definition and more open-ended objectives.

Audit places fewer demands upon analytical techniques, requiring generally sound simple practice without resort to more complex techniques. There are some very good reasons for this:

- the quality and quantity of data doesn't justify it
- the problem doesn't need it
- it wouldn't tell the target audience anything anyway.

Audit requires a focus and discipline which can be deleterious in research. There is evidence from early audit reports of a lack of structure and focus in studies tackled in the manner of research projects.

The Defect Analysis View

Crosby (1986) has pioneered the 'zero defect' view of quality in the manufacturing sector. This view emphasizes that many defects are preventable. By preventing defects, waste is reduced, leading to better quality and reduced costs. In this way, Crosby argues that quality improvement will be self-financing, whilst not improving will be prohibitively expensive in the long run.

The view focuses upon the negative (i.e. the absence of quality) because it is argued that this is easier to detect. In the medical context (Craddick & Bader, 1983) a US study of patients showed up to 20% had an adverse experience (a 'defect' in quality management parlance) during a hospital stay (Table 5.1). Other studies suggest even higher figures.

Table 5.1   'Defects' in hospital care

Defect	Occurrence
Re-infection	10%
Incomplete consent forms	4%
Cardiac/respiratory arrest	2%
Problems with intravenous cannulas/catheters	3%
Fall/slip	1%

Source: Craddick & Bader (1983) cited by Bennett & Walshe (1990)

A practical application of the identification and prevention of defects in the medical context is seen in 'occurrence screening'. In this approach, defects or 'adverse patient occurrences' are identified. The causes are then investigated and where possible eliminated. The advantages of this approach are:

- the ease of identifying defects
- that it facilitates the targeting of resources upon critical areas
- that identification of criteria for poor quality of care assists the clinician in the demonstration of proper care in the event of legal challenges.

The technique is of far greater importance in the US healthcare sector than in the UK, although significant pilot studies are under way in the UK (e.g. Bennett & Walshe, 1990). It is most attractive in those cultures where a key factor in the drive for better patient care is the fear of litigation. There is still currently significant cultural resistance amongst UK clinicians to a view of improving patient care based principally upon eliminating defects rather than making positive improvements.

Because of the importance of occurrence screening as a healthcare quality assurance mechanism in its own right outside the UK, we shall return to it in more detail in Chapter 7.

The Information Management View

Each of the views outlined thus far dominates a particular sector of healthcare. Managers and political leaders in the UK clearly see clinical audit as a quality assurance *process* and emphasize process improvement. Clinicians often adversarial to the management perspective, see clinical audit as part of their *research-based* traditions. In a culture where litigation is a major concern, such as the US healthcare industry, the *defect analysis* view will tend to dominate.

Each of these views brings particular assumptions and vices with it. The author proposes an alternative view based upon *information* to complement the other views. As with all views it comes from the author's own perspective and prejudices. This view is based upon the proposition that clinical audit, or indeed any quality mechanism in healthcare, depends crucially upon information and may be viewed as an information management problem. This view is intended to enrich our understanding of clinical audit and not to supplant any of the other views.

It is proposed because it may offer some or all of the following benefits:

- freedom from a prescriptive medical viewpoint
- neutrality in the clinical/managerial spectrum
- an emphasis upon improvement rather than defects
- facilitation of systematic data collection and analysis.

In this view, the process of clinical audit is seen in terms of information requirements. Clinical audit becomes a process of:

- establishing information needs
- gathering the required information
- analysing the information
- using the analysis results to inform and facilitate change in practice.

Information management encourages the establishment of clear aims and objectives. This assists clinicians in distinguishing research from audit. The view fits well with the use of computer technology to assist in data collection, processing and storage. The close relationship between computers and clinical audit will be examined in the next section.

5.4   THE ROLE OF COMPUTERS IN CLINICAL AUDIT

In the UK, audit has been introduced alongside many other management reforms. These reforms have all depended upon greater use of information and have led to an increased use in computer technology within the NHS. For example, in the primary healthcare sector computerization amongst family doctors has risen dramatically since 1985 (Fig. 5.4).

Computers offer many advantages to the auditor. Principally, they offer a convenient method to enter, store and process data. However, they should also increase reliability of analysis as well as convenience. The hackneyed expression 'garbage in, garbage out' is still true. Computers will generally analyse correctly and consistently the data they are given.

Nor does computerization have to be expensive. One of the best software packages available for most small-scale audit is Epi Info (Dean et al, 1995). Epi Info was developed as a tool for epidemiology by the World Health Organization and the Centers for Disease Control and Prevention. It is available free and may be copied without charge. Additionally, it does not require expensive computer hardware, running happily on computers regarded as obsolete by many. Its main disadvantage is its simple text-based user interface which is offputting to some users. The author has

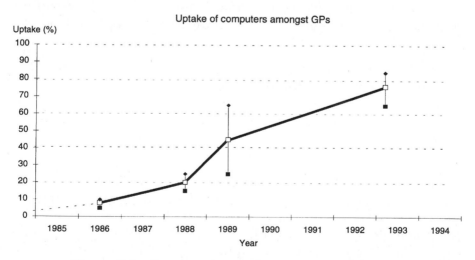

Figure 5.4   Computerization by general practitioners

discussed its use as an audit tool elsewhere (Gillies, 1994) and provided a practical guide to its use in clinical audit (Gillies, 1995).

In order to assess the impact of computerization upon clinical audit, we shall consider data collection, data storage and data analysis.

Data Collection

In order to assess the impact of computers upon the quality of data collection it is necessary to consider the process as an information chain. Table 5.2 lists the historical data sources most commonly used for clinical audit.

For the purpose of considering the quality of data collection we may classify data sources according to whether they are computer-based or paper-based and whether or not they are verifiable (Table 5.3).

The desirable characteristics for high-quality data collection are verifiable sources and a minimum number of data exchanges involving human action to minimize errors of transcription.

Studies based upon historical case notes are the least reliable. They are not verifiable and use human transcription to transfer data from paper records into electronic form on the computer. One way to improve on this is to use verifiable historical data sources when appropriate, such as X-ray films.

Where data are gathered contemporaneously through interview or questionnaire, there is the possibility of verification of data.

Table 5.2 Data sources for clinical audit (after Hunt and Legg, 1994)

Source type	Examples of specific sources
Registers	Cancer registry, diagnostic index, child health registers
Departmental records	Appointment books, pharmacy, theatre books
Professional notes	District nursing notes, ward kardex
Computer-based	Korner data, PAS, case mix system

Table 5.3   Data source classification for clinical audit
(after Gillies, 1995)

Source type	Examples
Historical physical	Historical paper-based patient records
Contemporary physical	Interview transcripts, questionnaire surveys
Historical verifiable physical	X-ray images
Direct electronic collection	Computer analysis of laboratory tests
Personal computer-based	Comparative data from previous audit
Mainframe computer-based	Korner data, PAS, case mix system

Normally, however, the technique is still prone to human transcription errors. Where questionnaires are used it may be possible to automate data compilation.

Table 5.4 summarizes the characteristics of the different data collection routes.

However, the computer can do more to improve data collection by protecting the data at the point of entry. Two types of data errors may be identified. They may be described as possible but incorrect and impossible values. The latter are easier to protect against. For example, if there are five possible responses coded 1 to 5, most computer systems will allow you to limit values entered for that field to 1, 2, 3, 4 or 5.

The second type of error is more tricky. In this case, an incorrect value between 1 and 5 is entered. This can only be protected by

Table 5.4   The quality of the different techniques

Source type	Availability	Verification	Transit errors
Historical physical	Good	Poor	Poor
Contemporary physical	Good	Good	Poor
Historical verifiable physical	Poor	Good	Poor
Direct electronic collection	Poor	Good	Good
Personal computer-based	OK	Poor	Good/OK
Mainframe computer-based	OK	Poor	OK

duplication of data entry. Again computer systems can help by providing easy ways to compare two versions of the same data file and identifying discrepancies.

To illustrate how effective this can be, imagine a dataset of 100 records each with 50 fields and a random data error rate of 2%. From this data one would predict that there would be 10 errors in the dataset after data entry. If data entry is repeated, then there will be a similar number of errors in the new dataset. However, the chances of those errors falling in one or more of the same fields is 0.04%.

Data Storage

The main advantage offered by the computer in terms of data storage is the convenience with which vast amounts of data can be stored. With proper backup procedures, computers can reliably store huge amounts of information for instant retrieval.

Data Analysis

Computers offer significant advantages in terms of data analysis. Even simple systems such as Epi, available without charge, can carry out chi-squared tests, sort data, stratify data and produce graphs.

However, the influence of the computer is not all good. The computer has had a negative impact as well, although usually this is implicit rather than explicit.

Consider, for example, data analysis. The computer will reliably carry out numerical analysis, but without enough knowledge to make correct use of the figures, this can be unhelpful.

An illustration of the dangers may be seen in an example from structural engineering, where stress analysis programmes were simplified to enable novice engineers to carry out complex calculations without specialist knowledge. Without the ability to interpret the figures critically, one such novice designed a concrete walkway using a literal interpretation of the figures. The walkway collapsed with fatal consequences. Whilst most difficulties will be of a lesser order, there are still dangers arising from uncritical interpretation of figures.

Even more insidious is the effect that computers have upon the audit cycle. Use of a computer focuses attention upon the initial stages of the audit cycle. This can exacerbate the tendency not to complete the audit cycle, and hence not to improve patient care.

5.5   STRENGTHS AND WEAKNESSES OF CLINICAL AUDIT

This section considers clinical audit as envisaged in an ideal form. The next chapter considers how far practice in one region meets the ideal.

The purpose of clinical audit is to assist in the management of patient care and to identify problems and to facilitate improvement. Clinical audit differs from other forms of audit in a number of key ways:

- It is perceived to be about a process of improvement rather than a snapshot of current performance.
- It is carried out at different levels within the organization, often initiated by local practitioners at their own level.
- It is not an overall process of quality assurance imposed from outside in the way that, for example, inspection of education is carried out.

The local control and ownership of audit is a direct consequence of the NHS reforms. From April 1995, financial responsibility for audit rests with the local trusts and districts (the purchasers in the NHS internal market). They are now able to target audit expenditure to the areas they wish.

This has a number of clear advantages in terms of user involvement and ownership. It greatly increases the enthusiasm of the practitioners for the process who perceive it as helpful in general rather than authoritarian.

The Weaknesses of Clinical Audit

The ideal form of clinical audit proposed by the White Paper is in fact far from ideal as a quality management procedure. Many of the limitations, however, may still reflect the fact that clinical audit is an optimal solution, a trade-off between two conflicting goals.

For example, in order to facilitate change, it is essential to establish local ownership and direction of projects. However, this reduces the effectiveness of audit as a tool for management. Many Regional Health Authorities have no central records of the number and nature of audits carried out. Local control implies a lack of central control. This changes the role of audit to a tool which feeds into operational management rather than strategic management. There is thus an inherent trade-off between local control and strategic effectiveness.

Another conflict may be seen in the focus of an audit. It has been stated that audits should be focused, not open-ended as in research. However, it is also suggested that audits should deal in underlying causes, not symptoms if real improvements are to achieved. This may not be possible if the approach adopted is too focused.

The use of computers has already highlighted the danger of too much focus on data collection and analysis at the expense of implemented change. At the same time, poor data will fail to deliver real improvement in practice.

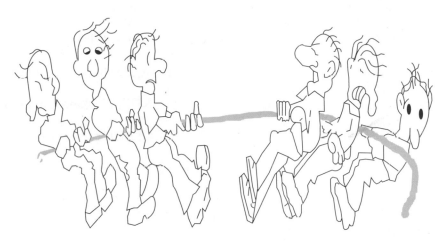

Strategic significance		Local ownership
Focus	V.	Underlying causes
Emphasis upon quality of data		Emphasis upon implementing change
Firefighting activity		Devoting time to long term improvement

Figure 5.5   Conflicts within clinical audit

Finally, there is the ultimate tension of best use of resources. If a doctor is overloaded, how far are you justified in increasing the problem by reducing the doctor's time to see patients by involving him or her in an audit to try to identify root causes of the problem?

The different views outlined above may be identified as having different positions on the conflicting desirable features. However, in addition to the inherent constraints detailed here, clinical audit as implemented still has considerable limitations as a practical technique. We shall explore these in the next chapter.

5.6   REFERENCES

Bennett, J. & Walshe, K. (1990) Occurrence screening as a method of audit. *British Medical Journal*, **300**, 1248–52.

Craddick, J. W. & Bader, B. (1983) *Medical Management Analysis: A Systematic Approach to Quality Assurance and Risk Management*. Auburn, CA: Joyce W. Craddick.

Crosby, P. B. (1986) *Quality is Free*. Maidenhead: McGraw-Hill.

Dean, J. A., Dean, A. G., Coulombie, D., Smith, D. C., Brendel, K. A. & Arner, T. G. (1995) *Epi Info Version 6: A Word-Processing, Database and Statistics Program for Epidemiology on Microcomputers*. Atlanta, GE: Centers for Disease Control and Prevention (available from USD Inc., 2075A West Park Place, Stone Mountain, GA 30087, USA; fax +404-469-0681).

Deming, W. E. (1986) *Out of the Crisis*. Cambridge, MA: MIT Center for Advanced Engineering.

Department of Health (1989) *Medical Audit* (NHS Working Paper 6). London: HMSO.

Garvin, D. (1984) What does quality mean? *Sloan Management Review*, **4**, 125–31.

Gillies, A. C. (1994) On the usability of software for medical audit. *Auditorium*, **3**(1), 14–20.

Gillies, A. C. (1995) *Information Management for Medical Audit: A Handbook*. Oxford University Postgraduate Medical Education and Training Department.

Hunt, V. & Legg, F. (1994) *Clinical Audit: A Basic Introduction*. Oxford University: Regional Postgraduate Medical Education & Training Office.

Juran, J. M. (1979) *Quality Control Handbook*, 3rd edn. Maidenhead: McGraw-Hill.

CHAPTER 6

The State of Clinical Audit: Experiences from the Oxford and Four Counties Region

with Nicola Ellis*

6.1   CHAPTER SUMMARY

This chapter examines the current practice of clinical audit within one region to consider how far in practice the purpose of audit to improve patient care is being realized.

The authors present the findings of a survey of published audit activity within the Oxford region of the UK (Ellis, 1995). The results indicate that there is some way to go before audit achieves its stated goal of directly improving patient care in all cases.

6.2   THE RESEARCH METHOD

The Oxford and Four Counties region is one of eight health regions formed after the 1993 reorganization within the UK National Health Service. This chapter reports findings from a

*The principal author would like to thank Nicola Ellis, Researcher, Information Management Research Group, for her help with this chapter, and acknowledge the assistance of the Oxford region in this study.

Table 6.1   The data entry form used in the study

SECTION A: What?

A1   What is the audit concerned with?

A2   Specialty?

A3   What level of audit is it?
1.   Resource based – quantity and type of resources available
2.   Process – what is done to the patient
3.   Outcome – results of clinical intervention
4.   Resource & Process
5.   Process & Outcome
6.   Resource & Outcome
7.   Process, Resource & Outcome

SECTION B: WHY?

B1   Why was it being carried out?
1.   Frequency of topic
2.   High risk area
3.   Known problem area
4.   High cost area
5.   Wide variation in clinical practice
6.   Local clinical anxiety
7.   Maximization of benefits
8.   Follow-up audits
9.   Other

SECTION C: When?

C1   When was it carried out?

SECTION D: Who?

D1   Who participated in/led the audit?

SECTION E: How?

E1   How was it carried out? Method?
1.   Retrospective review
2.   Questionnaire/survey
3.   Retrospective review and questionnaire/survey
4.   Other method

E2   Use of performance indicators? Which?

E3   Use of outcome measures? Which?

E4   How was it being controlled?

E5   Resources used?

E6   Sampling procedures used? Which?

Table 6.1   (continued)

E7   Method of data collection?
1.   Historical paper verifiable
2.   Historical paper case notes
3.   Historical electronic
4.   Live data questionnaire
5.   Other data

SECTION F: Results

F1   Improvement in care?
1.   direct improvement in care
2.   Indirect improvement in care
3.   No apparent improvement in care
F2   Implementation of changes?
F3   Re-audit/follow-up planned?
F4   Feedback of information?
F5   Standards set?
F6   Action taken?
1.   Publication and dissemination other than *Auditorium*
2.   Application of resources
3.   Remedial action
4.   Other action

study of clinical audit practice within this region and, prior to its formation, in the smaller Oxford region.

The study examined in detail a range of published audits, taken from the *Auditorium* journal since its inception in 1992 (Volumes 1:1–4:1). A standard data collection form (Table 6.1) was constructed to aid the investigation. Each audit dissemination was then taken in turn and examined with all pertinent data being extracted. The data gleaned was then keyed into Epi Info (Dean et al, 1995) and statistical analysis undertaken.

6.3   THE SAMPLE OF AUDITS STUDIED

The sample included audits from a wide range of clinical specialties, recorded in Table 6.2. The sample contained a range of problem types, classified as:

Table 6.2   Clinical specialities represented within the study

Speciality	Number of audits
Psychiatry	16
General surgery	11
Anaesthetics	7
A&E, gynaecology & obstetrics, orthopaedics	5
Paediatrics	4
Dermatology, gastroenterology, general medicine, ITU, ophthalmology, pathology, radiography	14
A&E/paediatrics, cardiology, community care, general practice, gerontology, health services research, neurophysiology, neuropsychology, orthodontics, paediatrics/G&O, pharmacology/ hospital management	18
Total	78

- *Resource-based:* to investigate the quantity and type of resources available
- *Patient-based:* to investigate actions concerning patients
- *Clinical-based:* to investigate the outcomes from clinical interventions.

The cross-section of audits investigated in terms of problem types is shown in Table 6.3.

Table 6.3   Types of problem under investigation

Problem type(s)	Number of audits
Resource based	15
Process based	14
Outcome based	7
Process and outcome based	11
Resource and process based	10
Resource and outcome based	2
Process, resource and outcome based	19
Total	78

There are many reasons for an audit to be carried out, and this variety is well represented in the sample (Table 6.4). It was felt that the reasons could be effectively encompassed within the following nine classifications, which are based upon those devised by Hunt and Legg (1994), Baker and Presley (1990), Shaw (1989), and Rigby et al (1992).

- *Known problem area:* Is there a known problem in this area already?
- *Frequency of topic:* Are large numbers of patients treated?
- *High risk:* The need to assess risk potential, or consequence of, patients undergoing a high risk procedure.
- *High cost area:* Are expensive procedures carried out inappropriately?
- *Wide variation in clinical practice.*
- *Local clinical anxiety.*
- *Maximization of benefits.*
- *Follow-up audit:* Is the audit being carried out as a result of changes implemented after a previous audit in the same area?
- *Other:* Anything not encompassed by the above eight classifications.

The majority of audits (58%) were undertaken as a result of a known problem in the area of concern.

Table 6.4 Audits studied classified by purpose

Audit purpose	Number of audits
Known problem area	44
Local clinical anxiety	9
Maximization of benefits	7
High cost area	6
Wide variation in clinical practice	5
Follow-up audit	3
Frequency of topic	2
High risk area	1
Other	1
Total	*78*

The audits studied were published during the years 1992 to 1994. However, the publication date did not necessarily reflect the date of completion. Where this information was available, it was recorded (53 audits). The sample is drawn principally from audits completed in years 1991 to 1993, for which an approximately equal number of audits is included (Table 6.5).

The sample contained a wide range of projects of varying durations. The distribution of durations amongst the sample is shown in Fig. 6.1.

Table 6.5   Year audit projects completed

Year	Number of audits
1990 and earlier	5
1991	15
1992	17
1993	13
1994	3
Total	53

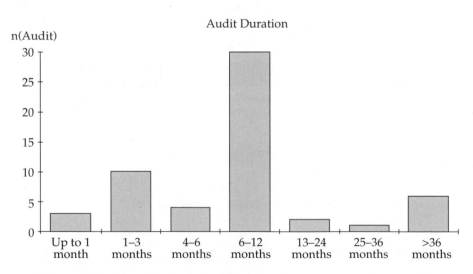

Figure 6.1   Distribution of audit durations amongst the sample

6.4   FINDINGS

The study set out to answer a series of questions.

Who is Involved in Audit?

The study showed that most audits are led by clinicians, confirming the local control and ownership of audit. Table 6.6 shows who was listed as authors of the published findings.

How is Audit Carried Out?

Four distinct approaches were identified within the sample:

* retrospective review
* questionnaire survey
* interview
* checklist.

The results are shown in Fig. 6.2. The majority of audits (58%)

Table 6.6   Personnel leading or playing a major part in audits

Personnel	Number of audits
Consultant	53
Registrar	26
Senior registrar	22
Audit staff	19
Nursing staff	13
SHO	12
GP	5
Researcher	5
Other	3
Lecturer/reader	2
Admin. assistant, anaesthetist, deputy director, multidisciplinary team, paediatric health visitor, pharmacist, psychiatrist, quality manager, statistician	1
Total	161

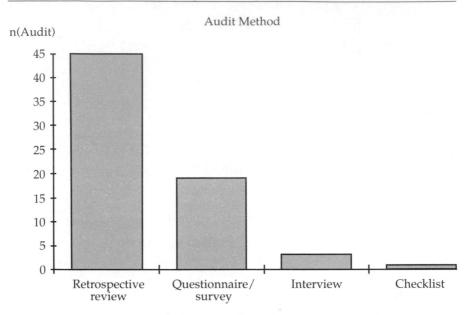

Figure 6.2   Single method used to carry out audit

utilized retrospective review as the audit method. The vast majority of audits (87%) used a single method, whilst 10 used a combination of methods to improve their data collection (Fig. 6.3).

What Measurement Techniques Were Employed?

In only five cases (6%) were performance indicators used, and in only seven cases (9%) were outcome measures used. The measures are summarized in Table 6.7.

Which Sampling Procedures Were Used?

Eighty-three percent of audits used a census as their sampling procedure. This may be attributed to the fact that the target population was so tightly and explicitly defined that few patients could match the specified criteria. The full results are shown in Table 6.8.

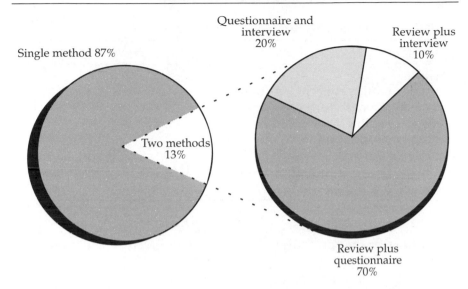

Figure 6.3   Combination method used to carry out audit

Table 6.7   Measures employed in audits studied

Performance indicators	Outcome measures
Comparison with NHLBI	Comparison with NHLBI
Level of self-administration achieved	Consultant rates
National ITU audit recommendations	Critical incident states
Triss methodology	Garden grades
Unit guidelines from previous audit	GHQ-30; symptomatic assessment/ SF36/Euroquol/TTO; Trauma chart

What Was the Method of Data Collection?

A range of methods was found either in combination or singly. These were classified as one of the following:

- historical verifiable, e.g. X-rays
- historical non-verifiable, e.g. case notes

Table 6.8   Sampling procedures employed

Sampling procedures	Number of audits
Census	65
Voluntary participation of census group	4
Voluntary response to census group	2
Random sampling (every 5th)	1
Random sampling within census group	1
Random selection	1
Voluntary response to questionnaires	1
Voluntary return of audit forms	1

- historical (non-verifiable) electronic, e.g. electronic patient records
- current written data, e.g. questionnaire survey
- current aural data, e.g. structured interview
- checklists.

Sixty-five audits used a single method of data collection whilst 13 used a combination of methods. The audits using a single data collection method are summarized in Fig. 6.4. The ten audits are summarized in Table 6.9.

How Many Audits Produced a Direct Improvement in the Quality of Patient Care?

The primary purpose of the study was to investigate whether an audit had resulted in a direct improvement in patient care and whether it had influenced future practice and proceedings. The study classified improvements in patient care resulting from the audit studies as direct, indirect or none:

- *Direct improvement:* An audit demonstrated a mechanism for directly improving the quality of patient care, usually as a result of changes being implemented as a result of the audit.
- *Indirect improvement:* Audits that implemented some form of feedback without a direct mechanism for improving care.
- *No apparent improvement:* Audits that did not appear to make any attempt to complete the audit cycle.

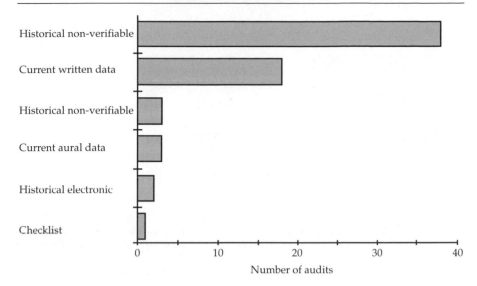

Figure 6.4 Audits employing a single method of data collection

Table 6.9 Summary of audits using combination data collection methods

Data collection methods	Number of audits
Historical verifiable (X-rays)/historical non-verifiable (case notes)	5
Historical non-verifiable (case notes)/current written data (questionnaire/survey)	4
Historical verifiable (X-rays)/current written data (questionnaire/survey)	1
Historical non-verifiable (case notes)/current aural data (structured interview)	1
Current written data (questionnaire/survey)/current aural data (structured interview)	1
Historical verifiable (X-rays)/current aural data (structured interview)	1

The findings are shown in Fig. 6.5.

It was also considered whether a re-audit or follow-up work had occurred or was planned. The mechanism for feeding back information from the audit was considered. In particular, the

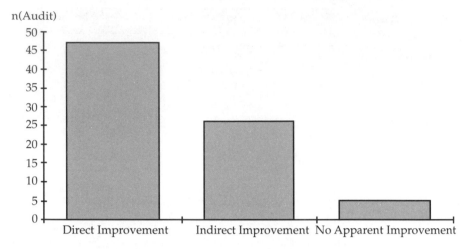

Figure 6.5   Improvements as a result of audits

study highlighted whether any standards had been set and whether action had been taken as a consequence of the audit (i.e. remedial action, publication and dissemination, application of resources). These factors are summarized in Table 6.10.

The audits in this study should represent good practice. However, only 60% produced an actual improvement in patient care and only 53% demonstrated a commitment to complete the audit cycle and re-audit to evaluate changes made.

Does Clinical Specialty Influence Audit Practice?

As the purpose of clinical audit is to improve practice, the study considered which external factors might influence the percentage of audits producing a direct improvement.

Table 6.10   Follow-up activities

Activity	Percentage of audits
Changes implemented	60%
Re-audit planned or carried out	47%
Results fed back	92%
Guidelines implemented	41%

The first factor to be considered is the clinical specialty. There are clear variations in the percentage of audits resulting in direct improvements, but the sample is too small for any firm conclusions when stratified by specialty. The results for the seven most common specialties in the sample are summarized in Fig. 6.6.

The study is ongoing. As the study develops, the samples will increase and it will be possible to investigate audit practice within specific disciplines.

Does the Type of Problem Tackled Affect the Likelihood of Direct Improvement?

The type of problem investigated had little effect on the outcome of the audit. Table 6.11, shows that the percentage of audits producing direct improvements is little affected.

When audits considering more than one type of problem are compared with those concerned with a single problem type, performance deteriorates. A chi-squared test was therefore carried out to investigate the hypothesis that multiple problem types caused a significant deterioration in performance ($\alpha = 0.05$). In

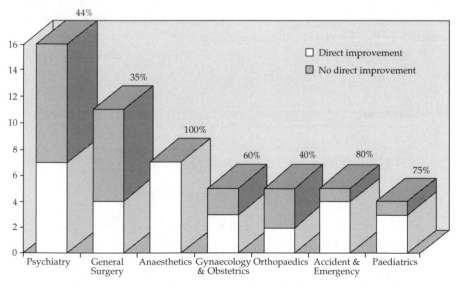

Figure 6.6   Direct improvements by clinical specialty

Table 6.11   Effect of problem type on audit practice

Problem type	Direct improvement	n
Clinical	59%	39
Patient	57%	54
Resource	57%	46

fact, a Fisher exact test gave a p-value of 0.2, failing to prove the hypothesis.

Does Audit Purpose Affect Audit Performance?

The purpose of the audit and its relationship with direct improvement in patient care was investigated. However, there is little evidence to support any relationship between these two variables, as shown in Table 6.12.

Is Audit Practice Improving?

Clinical audit practice in the UK is a relatively immature discipline. It therefore seems quite likely that performance is improving with time. This hypothesis is supported but not proven by Fig. 6.7. If we regard pre-1991 and 1994 as providing insufficient data, then there is an encouraging rising trend.

Table 6.12   Audit purpose and its impact on performance

Audit purpose	Direct	n
Known problem area	59%	44
Local clinical anxiety	56%	9
Maximization of benefits	57%	7
High cost area	33%	6
Wide variation in clinical practice	60%	5
Follow-up audit	100%	3
Frequency of topic	100%	2
High risk area	100%	1
Other	100%	1

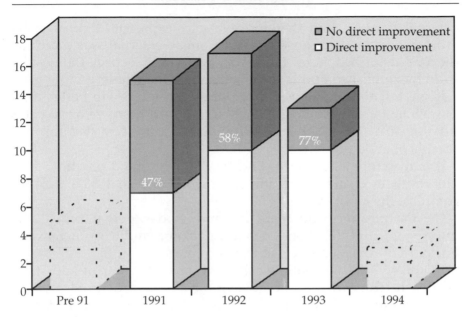

Figure 6.7   Improvements in practice over the years 1991–1993

As the study progresses this trend will be monitored to see whether the improvement over just a few years can be maintained.

6.5   CONCLUSIONS

The study relates to one region. The sample of published audits is not intended to be representative of the whole, but rather to represent a sample of good practice.

This can be tested by comparing the sample with the figures published by the Anglia and Oxford Regional Health Authority and NHS Executive (1994) pertaining to audits for the year 1993/ 1994. The annual report states that:

> In 1993/94 there were over 1500 audit projects carried out in the Oxford Region, of which 46% involved the development of standards or guidelines and 33% led to practice improvements.

The annual report is based upon self assessment rather than

external scrutiny, and therefore we may expect its figures to be more optimistic than those derived from an external study such as the one described here. However, we would expect the results from the published audits to be better than the whole.

If we test the hypothesis that published audits are better than the whole by constructing a chi-squared test, then we arrive at a p-value of 2×10^{-4}, which confirms our supposition that this is a sample of good practice.

It is therefore alarming to find that 40% of 'good practice' does not result in changes and improvements, and that 53% did not complete the audit cycle.

On the positive side there is some evidence that practice is improving, and that understanding about audit is increasing. Further improvements are, however, required.

It is likely that this will be achieved through a 'carrot and stick' approach. The carrot is the development of a structured method and computerized tool to facilitate good practice. This is the subject of ongoing research by the authors. The stick is the tighter control of resources allocated under the 'audit' label. Projects must demonstrate commitment to real improvements in care before money is provided.

6.6   REFERENCES

Anglia and Oxford RHA & NHS Executive (1994) *Anglia & Oxford Clinical Audit in the Hospital and Community Health Services: Annual Report 1993/94*. Oxford: AORHA/NHSE.

Baker, R. & Presley, P. (1990) *The Practice Audit Plan*. Bristol: Severn Faculty of the Royal College of General Practitioners.

Dean, J. A., Dean, A. G., Coulombie, D., Smith, D. C., Brendel, K. A. & Arner, T. G. (1995) *Epi Info Version 6: A Word-Processing, Database and Statistics Program for Epidemiology on Microcomputers*. Atlanta, GE: Centers for Disease Control and Prevention (available from USD Inc., 2075A West Park Place, Stone Mountain, GA 30087, USA; fax +404-469-0681).

Ellis, N. T. (1995) Audit of audit: a survey of audit practice in the four counties, Anglia and Oxford region. *Auditorium*, 4(2), 8–10.

Hunt, V. & Legg, F. (1994) *Clinical Audit: A Basic Introduction*. Oxford University: Regional Postgraduate Medical Education & Training Office.

Rigby, M., McBride, A. & Shiels, C. (1992) *Computers in Medical Audit.* London: University of Keele/West Midlands RHA/Royal Society of Medicine Services Ltd.

Shaw, C. D. (1989) *Medical Audit: A Hospital Handbook.* London: King's Fund Centre.

CHAPTER 7

Experience With Occurrence Screening

7.1 CHAPTER SUMMARY

This chapter describes the occurrence screening approach. This is probably the principal mechanism for improving patient care in the USA. The major differences in structure and culture of healthcare between the USA and UK make for an interesting comparison.

After describing the approach, the chapter considers some US experience and then examines in detail a case study illustrating the limited use that has been made of the approach in the UK.

The chapter concludes with a summary of the strengths and weaknesses of this technique.

7.2 OCCURRENCE SCREENING AS A QUALITY MANAGEMENT MECHANISM

It has already been suggested that the audit cycle has its roots in the classic process improvement ideas of Deming. Occurrence screening may be seen as the application in healthcare of Crosby's view of quality as 'zero defects', since it seeks to identify defects and eliminate them.

Occurrence screening techniques were developed in California in the 1970s (CMA/CHA, 1977). The technique was born out of a study into the level of claims for medical negligence. The study produced unremarkable findings, but the methods were refined and developed to become the Medical Management System of quality assurance.

The technique works by reviewing examples of patient care selected by trained staff using screening criteria. Where a case meets one or more of the criteria, it is sent for peer review. If the peer reviewer considers the case serious enough, they may bring it to a broader audience, usually a regular audit meeting.

The investigated cases can be built up to provide a database of instances which can then be used to evaluate trends and underlying causes with a view to eliminating examples of poor care.

Philosophically, this approach is close to Crosby's idea of zero defects, which assumes that when all errors have been eliminated then quality has been achieved. This may be contrasted with process improvement where it is deemed that improvement is a continuing process. This will be further explored at the end of the chapter.

7.3   EXPERIENCE WITH OCCURRENCE SCREENING IN THE USA

Occurrence screening forms a significant part of the US quality assurance process. Carlow (1988) cites the following facts:

- It is recommended by the American College of Surgeons and the American College of Anesthesiology.
- It is employed in over 200 hospitals.
- It is mandatory in all Department of Defense hospitals.
- It has been used by all professional review organizations since 1986.
- It forms the basis of clinical indicators developed by the Joint Commission for the Accreditation of Health Care Organizations (Shaw, 1988).

There have been a number of studies to evaluate the effectiveness of the technique. Panniers & Newlander (1986) studied 426 myocardial infarction patients and concluded that the screening criteria used were both valid and reliable. This finding was reinforced by a more recent study due to Brennan and colleagues

(1989, 1990). This was concerned with adverse events occurring during hospitalization, varying from infections to a slip or a fall or life-threatening clinical incidents such as cardiac arrest. The study used multiple reviews of 360 hospital patient records and again concluded that the results of the screening process were valid and reliable.

However, other authors such as Schumacher et al (1987) have observed inconsistencies between different observers. This study was based upon 752 patients with a wide range of diagnoses.

Whilst proponents are enthusiastic about the benefits, it is reasonable to conclude that care is needed in the application of the technique, as with any other method.

However, it should also be noted that occurrence screening is generally regarded as part of an overall effort to improve quality, rather than a method to replace all others. In such form, it is likely to make a useful contribution to the overall effort to improve patient care.

7.4   EXPERIENCE WITH OCCURRENCE SCREENING IN THE UK

Occurrence screening is not prevalent in the UK. The information systems of UK hospitals are not designed to record instances of adverse patient occurrences. Where such incidences are recorded it is often done on an *ad hoc* basis, and does not provide a suitable basis for occurrence screening.

Occurrence screening has recently been piloted at a number of sites, including the Royal Sussex County Hospital, Brighton. We shall consider this as a case study.

Occurrence Screening at the Royal Sussex County Hospital

This project was a pilot sponsored by the Department of Health and carried out by Brighton Health Authority and CASPE Research. The project was established with four objectives:

- to investigate the reliability and validity of the occurrence screening technique as a measure of hospital care

- to encourage the development of peer review mechanisms within the hospital medical and nursing staff
- to establish whether the mechanisms established facilitate changes in clinical practice
- to establish benchmarks to identify the cost-effectiveness (or otherwise) of occurrence screening.

The research team felt that existing models of peer review, developed within the North American context, were not completely appropriate for the UK, so a modified procedure was developed, as shown in Fig. 7.1.

The main study was preceded by a pilot study at the smaller Hove Hospital, in 1988. It was used as a feasibility study for the main project. Eleven criteria were selected for use from American studies. They were first translated into UK English, with particular care taken with terminology. Four further criteria were added locally. The criteria used were:

- readmission with clinical complications arising from earlier admission
- consent for operation
- unplanned return to theatre
- patient transfused
- hospital-acquired infection
- cardiac or respiratory arrest
- hospital incident
  - accident
  - intravenous catheter problem
  - skin problems (e.g. bedsores)
  - equipment failure
  - other
- transfer to special care unit
- transfer to other hospital
- death
- patient and/or family dissatisfaction
- resuscitation category noted
- discharge note
- discharge summary
- property form signed.

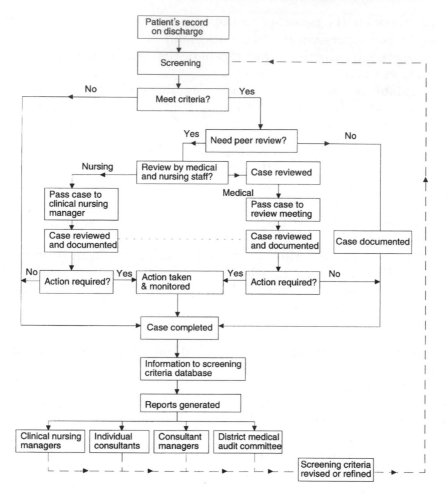

Figure 7.1   Review procedure employed at the Royal Sussex County Hospital (after Bennett & Walshe, 1990)

In the pilot, the notes were screened by a medical administrator. A sample was checked by a doctor, who found no problems with the screening. It was found that screening was most efficient when carried out soon after discharge. In such circumstances, each record took less than 10 minutes to screen in over 90% of cases.

The pilot indicated an adverse experience occurrence rate of 22%. This is comparable with American studies and was assumed to be indicative of the rate that could be anticipated for the main study. Whilst some problems were experienced, the pilot demonstrated the feasibility of the larger study in the British context.

The main project used three staff, all qualified nurses, to screen over 13 000 patient records between February 1990 and April 1992. The patients were drawn from 12 specialties.

The project surveyed 150 clinicians to establish whether the procedure was valid from a content viewpoint. The project database was evaluated to test construct validity. The reliability of the screening process, queried in some American studies, was tested by parallel screening studies to assess consistency between different personnel, and by rescreening studies to assess individuals over time. The project found the measure to be valid and reliable.

The project evaluated the usefulness of reports provided to clinicians in a wide variety of formats and styles, e.g. graphical, tabular, lists. The clinicians reported that there was a danger of information overload. As a consequence, the most useful reports were found to be concise and focused upon specific issues.

The effect upon practice is more difficult to evaluate within the life of the project. However, some improvements were noted in the availability of equipment and the quality of patient records. This was observed through a reduction in adverse event rates with respect to these items.

The final aim concerned the cost-effectiveness of the technique. Four cost areas were defined:

- data collection
- data processing
- clinician involvement
- changes in practice.

As with the effect upon practice, some of these costs may be difficult to assess within a short project. However, the data collection time was measured at an average of 11 minutes and the cost of data entry and collection was estimated to be around £3.50.

The project was successful in evaluating the technique in a UK context and provided encouraging results for further adoption in the NHS context.

7.5   STRENGTHS AND WEAKNESSES OF OCCURRENCE SCREENING

Occurrence screening was born out of work carried out to reduce malpractice suits. It has at its heart a view that quality is equivalent to zero defects. There are several factors that have encouraged its adoption within the US medical system:

- It was developed within that system.
- It is well suited to identifying potential malpractice, which might lead to a malpractice suit.
- The importance of litigation as a cultural factor in the American medical system encourages a zero defect view of quality.

In other countries, these factors are less positive in favouring occurrence screening. Litigation culture is less dominant. As fear of litigation rises, then occurrence screening may become more popular.

At the heart of any comparison of occurrence screening with quality methods based upon process improvement, is the difference in views of quality that the methods are designed to satisfy. Occurrence screening is derived from a technique to reduce malpractice suits. Therefore, it is designed to reduce what are called non-conformances in quality terminology, which could lead to a malpractice suit.

By contrast, process improvement techniques as enshrined within clinical audit are intended to improve patient care. This may appear to be the same thing, and indeed it will often prove to be so. However, there are specific cases where the doctors' and patients' best interests may not be the same.

Consider, for example, the delivery of children. Caesarean section births are more risky for the patient than birth canal deliveries. However, there is a lower risk to the doctor associated with the caesarean delivery, since it is easier to prove that all precautions have been taken. Therefore, at a time when it was known that caesarean deliveries were more risky to the patient their use was still growing in the USA. This trend was only halted by a series of lawsuits alleging that a caesarean procedure had been adopted against the patients' interests.

In essence, the difference between process improvement and

occurrence screening is that occurrence screening seeks to establish a level of satisfactory performance, whereas process improvement assumes that there is always room for improvement.

To explore the implications of this, consider perinatal mortality data from five different countries since 1970 (see Fig. 7.2). The figures themselves are shown in Table 7.1.

The figures illustrate that all these countries have improved the quality of patient care in this area. They illustrate the relative nature of quality. In 1970, patient care in the Netherlands was clearly better than anywhere else. The UK was better than all but the Netherlands. Austria and Malta were about the same and Romania was considerably worse than any of the Western nations.

Although there have been improvements in all countries since then, it is not possible to set an acceptable level of performance above zero. Process improvement would argue that there is

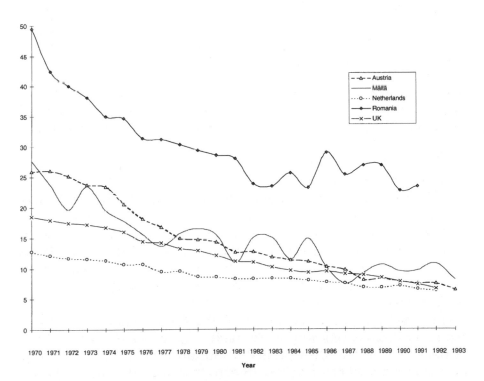

Figure 7.2 Perinatal mortality rate per 1000 births (WHO, 1994)

Table 7.1   Perinatal mortality data since 1970 (WHO, 1994)

Year	Austria	Malta	Netherlands	Romania	UK
1970	25.89	27.66	12.75	49.43	18.49
1971	26.10	23.73	12.14	42.39	17.93
1972	25.20	19.68	11.70	40.00	17.50
1973	23.78	23.44	11.53	38.14	17.23
1974	23.45	19.50	11.31	34.97	16.76
1975	20.54	17.82	10.65	34.67	16.04
1976	18.22	15.63	10.70	31.36	14.47
1977	16.81	13.64	9.52	31.15	14.16
1978	14.98	15.78	9.58	30.27	13.26
1979	14.75	16.49	8.71	29.31	12.90
1980	14.34	15.53	8.59	28.56	12.10
1981	12.66	10.96	8.30	28.03	11.16
1982	12.79	15.05	8.29	23.88	10.98
1983	11.88	15.04	8.41	23.41	10.20
1984	11.41	11.49	8.36	25.62	9.61
1985	11.17	14.92	8.04	23.21	9.36
1986	10.27	10.10	7.77	28.91	9.51
1987	9.83	7.53	7.60	25.37	9.12
1988	8.13	9.22	6.83	26.90	8.97
1989	8.31	10.57	6.78	26.91	8.42
1990	7.84	9.5	7.08	22.73	7.85
1991	7.48	9.62	6.50	23.35	7.35
1992	7.53	10.78	6.29	No data	6.58
1993	6.49	8.16	No data	No data	No data

always room for improvement and even the Netherlands has continually improved performance.

However, as improvements are wrought, there is a convergence of performance which suggests that it may not be possible to reduce perinatal mortality much below 6 per 1000 births. This reinforces a view that there is an acceptable practical limit of performance.

This does not allow for the possibility that a change in procedure or resource allocation may make a qualitative improvement in performance. Swedish perinatal mortality for 1992 is found to be 4.5 per 1000 births. For the 18 countries recorded in the WHO European database with data for 1991, there is found to be no correlation ($r = -0.56$) between simple expenditure *per capita* on healthcare and perinatal mortality. This would seem to encourage the view that other nations could still improve performance by up to 25% by changes in either healthcare practice or other factors such as environment or diet.

In practice, the distinction between methods based upon the audit cycle and occurrence screening is not always clear-cut. For example, many audits seek to improve practice by implementing clinical guidelines and standards. These can result in a view of quality which assumes that if guidelines are being met, then quality is being delivered. This view equates to a 'zero defects' (Crosby) or manufacturing (Garvin) view of quality normally associated with occurrence screening techniques rather than a process improvement view. The above data indicate that even when performance may be relatively good, there is still room for improvement. This may be a situation revealing few apparent defects or adverse events.

Similarly, many defects identified through occurrence screening have resulted in improvements. If there is a commitment to revisit the same area, then the process may be viewed as a stepwise improvement process.

7.6 REFERENCES

Bennett, J. & Walshe, K. (1990) Occurrence screening as a method of audit. *British Medical Journal*, **300**, 1248–52.

Brennan, T. A., Localio, R. J. & Laird, N. L. (1989) Reliability and validity of judgements concerning adverse events suffered by hospitalised patients. *Medical Care*, **27**, 1148–58.

Brennan, T. A., Localio, R. J. & Leape, L. L. (1990) Identification of adverse events occurring during hospitalisation. *Annals of Internal Medicine*, **112**, 221–6.

California Medical Association and California Hospital Association (1977) *Report on the Medical Insurance Feasibility Study*. San Francisco: Sutter Publications.

Carlow, D. (1988) Occurrence screening can improve QA programs. *Dimensions Health Service*, **65**, 20–2.

Panniers, T. L. & Newlander, J. (1986) The adverse patient occurrences inventory: validity, reliability and implications. *Quality Review Bulletin*, **12**, 311–15.

Schumacher, D. N., Parker, B. & Kofie, V. (1987) Severity of illness index and the adverse patient occurrence index: a reliability study and policy implications. *Medical Care*, **25**, 695–704.

Shaw, C. D. (1988) Clinical outcome indicators. *Health Trends*, **21**, 37–40.

World Health Organization (1994) *Health for All Database*, World Wide Web. Geneva: WHO.

CHAPTER 8

Development and Use of Clinical Outcome/ Performance Indicators

Jan Barnsley, Louise Lemieux-Charles, G. Ross Barker*

8.1 CHAPTER SUMMARY

This chapter is based on practical experience within the Canadian healthcare system. It describes the development and use of performance indicators within hospitals in Ontario, Canada.

The chapter describes a study designed to investigate whether performance indicators can assist clinicians and managers in the provision of healthcare. It outlines the methods used in the investigation and considers the findings.

8.2 BACKGROUND

During the past decade, the quality of care provided by healthcare organizations has received increasing attention from government, providers and consumers in North America. Before the

---

*The principal author wishes to thank the Canadian authors for this chapter and their valued contribution.

mid-eighties, quality-related issues, such as effectiveness and appropriateness of care, were subordinate to concerns for efficiency and cost containment. Many changes were generated to improve efficiency; however, assessment of the impact of these changes on aspects of quality did not necessarily ensue. There followed a number of years during which quality considerations became an impetus for change rather than a mere afterthought. However, continued and more dramatic cutbacks have raised concerns regarding the impact of reduced resources, and the attending structural changes on quality of care.

These concerns, combined with the belief that efficiency and effectiveness are both achievable in a well managed system, have led to—or at least coincided with—the advent of innovative approaches to measuring provider performance and to managing the provision of healthcare to enhance quality. Noteworthy is the shift from a dependence on structure and process measures of quality to the development and use of outcome measures (Lohr, 1988; O'Leary, 1993; Reinertsen, 1993). Donabedian (1980) introduced the conceptual framework of structure, process and outcome to support quality assurance activities. At first, structural measures (e.g. adequacy of facilities, equipment, personnel) and process measures (e.g. adequacy of clinical procedures) provided the basis for performance assessment. The logic was that if structure and process standards were met, high quality care and good outcomes would be guaranteed. However, the links between structure and process factors and patient outcomes are not always clear and adherence to standards does not always result in good outcomes. This realization, combined with the continuous quality improvement perspective which emphasizes a dynamic approach to ensuring quality of care rather than the more static adherence to standards, encouraged the development of outcome-based performance measures. Outcome measures gain additional importance given ongoing structural changes (mergers, alliances, re-engineering, downsizing) and process changes (reduced length of stay, increased same day procedures) that are, at least in part, encouraged/dictated by financial exigencies.

Clinical outcome indicators are measurable elements in the outcome of care which suggest one or more dimensions of quality of care. As with clinical performance measures, generally, clinical outcome indicators estimate the extent to which a health care provider delivers clinical services that are appropriate for each patient's condition; provides them safely, competently, and in an appropriate time frame. (Palmer, 1996.)

To be useful the outcomes upon which the indicators are based must link to structures and processes that can be altered by the providers of care (Bernstein and Hilborne, 1993; Davies et al, 1994). There are different types of outcome measures: those that measure actual patient functional status, well-being or satisfaction with care, and those that assess financial cost to the patient or to the healthcare system. In addition, some outcome measures are used to assess patient status during and immediately following inpatient care, while others assess the long-term health status of patients following their contact with a provider. Outcome measures can be applied across a wide range of diagnoses or procedures—for example, unplanned return to the operating room. Alternatively they can be disease-specific or procedure-specific—for example, functional status following total hip replacement. Finally, there are outcome measures that focus on adverse events (morbidity, mortality) and those that measure achievement of positive outcomes (e.g. vaginal birth after caesarean section).

To date, clinical outcome indicators have played a minor role in clinical care evaluation. The limited use of clinical outcome indicators is not surprising; their development demands time and effort which are in short supply in most healthcare facilities. Nevertheless, properly constructed indicators can point the direction to improved care processes, ultimately reducing the time and effort required to provide high quality care.

This chapter describes a collaborative study by the Hospital Management Research Unit of the University of Toronto and the Ontario Council of Teaching Hospitals (OCOTH). It entailed the development of clinical outcome indicators, formulation of two sets of outcome indicator reports (hospital-specific and comparative), dissemination of the reports to teaching hospitals, and a follow-up survey to determine the perceived usefulness of the indicator reports and their actual use.

The purpose of the study was to determine:

(a) whether the specific set of clinical outcome indicators provide

useful information to managers and/or clinicians (i.e. physicians and nurses)
(b) whether indicator information is used and how it is used
(c) how to improve clinical outcome indicators.

8.3   METHODS

Selection of Clinical Outcome Indicators

Individual and group interviews were conducted in 18 teaching hospitals in the province of Ontario, Canada. A staff member in each hospital, appointed by the chief executive officer to act as the liaison between the hospital and the project, identified hospital staff to be interviewed by the research team.

Over 100 staff, including physicians, nurses, health records personnel, and middle and senior managers, took part in interviews to assist in identifying clinical performance indicators that were considered both relevant to their work and feasible in terms of data collection. Based upon these interviews, five sets of indicators were selected, as shown in Table 8.1.

- *Unplanned readmission to hospital* is the unplanned readmission to the index hospital via the emergency department for the same or related diagnosis within one month. It excludes alcohol or drug addiction-related readmissions, AIDS-related readmissions, obstetric readmissions following discharge without delivery (e.g. false labour), readmissions for standard chemotherapy treatments without complications, and readmissions for standard dialysis treatment without complications.
- *Unplanned return to the operating room* is an unscheduled or

Table 8.1   Clinical outcome indicators selected for the study

Unplanned readmission to hospital
Unplanned return to the operating room
Unplanned inpatient admission from same-day surgery
Caesarean section
Low Apgar score in newborns

unexpected inpatient return to an operating room for complications or adverse outcomes that might be related to previous surgical procedures or care received during the same admission.

- *Unplanned inpatient admission from same-day surgery* is any patient admission to the same hospital directly from same-day surgery (i.e. transfer to inpatient status) which was not designated as planned and where there was no indication in the chart that the admission from same-day surgery was scheduled or expected.
- *Caesarean section* includes primary caesarean section, repeat caesarean section, with and without trial of labour, and vaginal birth after a previous caesarean section.
- *Low Apgar score in newborns* is an Apgar score of 6 or less, five minutes after delivery.

Data Collection

Special data collection was required for each of the indicator sets. This was accomplished through the efforts of the hospitals' medical records staff and the Canadian Institute for Health Information (CIHI) which collects standard discharge information from hospitals throughout Canada.

For an 18-month period, medical record staff coded non-standard data elements required to produce the indicators on special project lines provided on the CIHI forms. Non-standard data included: indication of whether readmissions, returns to the operating room, or inpatient admissions from same-day surgery were planned or unplanned, whether or not women with a previous caesarean section had an attempted vaginal birth prior to a repeat caesarean section, newborn Apgar scores, and the start and end time for surgical procedures. A detailed codebook was prepared and piloted by the research team prior to use by medical records staff for coding the special data elements. Coders had ongoing access to a member of the research team for help with coding problems.

A special edit was prepared for the new data elements by CIHI to check for errors and return problematic cases to the hospitals for correction. As well, a reabstraction of the non-standard data elements was conducted several months into the project to assess the reliability of the special data elements being collected for each indicator. The average percentage agreement across all hospitals between the coding by the medical records expert hired to do the reabstraction and the original coders was 98% for Apgar score, 94% for unplanned hospital readmission, 92% for trial of labour prior to a repeat caesarean section, 78% for unplanned inpatient admission from same-day surgery, and 63% for unplanned return to the operating room.

Preparation and Dissemination of Indicator Reports

Significant computer programming was required to prepare a method to adjust for patient morbidity. The Comorbidity Index developed by Charlson et al (1987), which is based on chronic diagnoses and age, was adapted to produce three morbidity classifications (mild, moderate, and severe). The morbidity adjustment was applied to three of the indicators—hospital readmission, inpatient admission from same-day surgery, and return to the operating room. The Comorbidity Index is not appropriate for use with newborns and obstetric patients.

Indicator data collected by the 18 hospitals between October 1992 and September 1993 were analysed and reported back to the hospitals. Decisions on the content and format of the indicator reports were guided by broad consultation with staff in each hospital and the Project Steering Committee. Two types of reports were prepared. The first contained indicator information specific to each hospital, and the second presented comparative information on all hospitals that provided required data on the particular indicators sets. Table 8.2 presents the number of hospitals providing data for each indicator.

Table 8.2 Number of hospitals providing data for each indicator

Unplanned readmission to hospital	17
Unplanned admission from same-day surgery	18
Unplanned return to the operating room	18
Caesarean section	13
Low Apgar score	13

The hospital-specific reports were extremely time-consuming to prepare as they provided information on diagnoses, diagnosis types (most responsible, primary, complication, comorbidity), procedures, dates of procedures, and most responsible physician for each indicator case. These reports were sent to all hospitals for the first quarter of the study period (October–December 1992) and, thereafter, were prepared by request only. Quarterly comparative reports were prepared and distributed to all hospitals for the entire one-year period. This chapter will present the results of the follow-up survey for the comparative reports only.

The comparative reports included tables and graphs for each outcome indicator rate (including numerator and denominator information) by hospital and by morbidity classification where appropriate. Ninety percent confidence intervals were calculated for hospital indicator rates as well as for the average indicator rates for all hospitals. The graphs enabled the reader to view the hospital-specific rates in relation to the group average. Reference notes regarding definitions, rate calculations and data limitations were attached to each set of indicator table and charts.

In the first quarterly comparative report, hospitals were represented by a unique letter code. Communication with the OCOTH council representatives through the Ontario Hospital Association, Speciality and Teaching Hospitals Division determined that hospitals were willing to be identified by name in the remaining comparative reports.

A copy of each indicator report was sent to the liaison person in each hospital with a request to communicate the contents of the reports or distribute the actual reports to the appropriate clinicians and managers. The identification of appropriate staff and the methods used to communicate the contents of the reports were left to the discretion of each hospital. The liaison person in each hospital was asked to provide us with the names of individuals who had access to the information in the reports. Seventeen of the 18 hospitals complied, providing us with a list of 247 staff names.

Follow-up Survey

Each staff member was sent an evaluation questionnaire which covered the following topics related to the comparative reports:

- whether the comparative reports were reviewed
- which sections dedicated to specific indicators were reviewed
- relevance of the information contained in the reports to the work of the respondent
- whether the information in the reports was used
- if used, how the information was used
- if not used, why the information was not used
- whether the hospital should continue to collect, report, and exchange the indicator information contained in the reports with other hospitals
- assessment of the format of the reports.

The questionnaire was pre-tested by two hospital liaisons and two other staff from two hospitals in Toronto. No substantive changes were required as a result of the pre-test. The package mailed to each potential respondent included a personally addressed letter of introduction, the questionnaire bearing a unique identification number, and a postage paid return envelope. Five weeks following the initial mailing, a follow-up questionnaire which was a shortened version of the initial questionnaire was mailed to all non-respondents. Completed questionnaires were received from 174 of the 247 possible respondents for a response rate of 70%. However, as shown in Table 8.3, not all respondents reviewed the information on all five indicators.

8.4   RESULTS

Of the 103 people who reported that they had reviewed at least one section of the comparative indicator reports, slightly less

Table 8.3   Number of respondents reviewing each section of the indicator report

Unplanned hospital readmission	95
Unplanned admission from same-day surgery	82
Unplanned return to the operating room	81
Caesarean section	60
Low Apgar score	57

than half, 44% ($n = 45$), used the information contained in the report; 56% ($n = 58$) had not used the indicator information (see Table 8.4).

Seventy-four percent of the 45 'users' presented the information at meetings and to committees, while 26% used the information to guide specific changes in policies and procedures. Those who did not use the information were asked to specify why they did not. Thirty-eight percent stated that lack of time prevented them from using the information, 22% said they were not sure how to use the information, and 31% were not sure that the information was reliable.

Table 8.5 presents responses to questions about the relevance of

Table 8.4 Proportion of respondents who used the information contained in the indicator reports

Used the information contained in the indicator reports for:	
presentation to meetings, further dissemination	74% (31/45)
specific changes to policies/procedures	26% (11/45)
Did not use the information contained in the indicator reports because:	
lack of time	38% (22/58)
not sure how to use the information	22% (13/58)
not sure data is reliable	31% (18/58)

Table 8.5 How relevant to your work is the indicator information contained in the comparative report?

	Moderately relevant	Very relevant
Unplanned hospital readmission	34% (32)	46% (44)
Inpatient admission from same-day surgery	20% (16)	53% (43)
Return to the operating room	23% (19)	53% (43)
Caesarean section	27% (16)	54% (32)
Low Apgar score	30% (9)	57% (17)

NB: The number of individuals responding to the indicator-specific questions varied across indicators the indicators to the respondent's work. Between 73% and 81% of respondents considered each indicator to be moderately or very relevant (as compared to 'slightly relevant' or 'not relevant').

Not surprisingly, in light of the level of relevance assigned to the indicators, between 70% and 94% of respondents wanted their hospital to continue to collect information on the various indicators and to continue to exchange indicator information with other teaching hospitals (see Table 8.6).

Finally, as shown in Table 8.7, over 85% of the 80 people responding to the question on report format indicated that the notes and definitions, the tables, and the graphs were moderately or very easy to understand.

In summary, the respondents were enthusiastic about the relevance and format of the indicator reports and thought the indicator data should continue to be gathered and exchanged.

Table 8.6   Would you like your hospital to continue to collect and exchange information with other teaching hospitals?

	'Yes' responses
Unplanned hospital readmission	88% (76)
Unplanned inpatient admission from same-day surgery	87% (65)
Unplanned return to the operating room	86.5% (64)
Caesarean section	94% (51)
Low Apgar score	79% (38)

NB: The number of individuals responding to the indicator-specific questions varied across indicators

Table 8.7   In the comparative indicator report, how easy was it to understand?

	'Moderate to very easy' responses
The notes and definitions	94% (75)
The table of rates	91% (73)
The graphs of rates	87.5% (70)

However, fewer than half actually used the information contained in the report for any purpose. Of those that did use the indicator reports, the majority used the information for 'passive' purposes of further dissemination at meetings while the minority actively applied the clinical indicator information to change policies or practices.

8.5   DISCUSSION AND CONCLUSIONS

Data collection, report preparation, dissemination, and follow-up were extremely labour-intensive in this project. The programming requirements and testing procedures took over a year to complete. If these activities were part of ongoing clinical outcome monitoring, additional resources would be required. However, the CIHI has expressed interest in revising the data collected in the discharge abstracts. If CIHI included the necessary data elements in their standard data collection and reporting, the hospitals could concentrate resources on effective dissemination and follow-up of the indicators in order to identify opportunities to improve structures and processes associated with the outcomes and to improve the indicators themselves.

As noted above, about one-third of respondents who did not use the indicator report information were not sure of the data reliability. There are a number of problems associated with hospital policies and practices that undermine the reliability of the indicators when used for comparative purposes.

- Some hospitals use ICD9 diagnostic codes while other hospitals use ICD9-CM. Fortunately a computer algorithm can be created to transform all codes to the less detailed ICD9 codes.
- Since reporting is not mandatory for all data elements in the CIHI abstract, hospitals vary in the reporting of optional items such as hospital readmission, anaesthesia technique, operating room identifier, and specialty/subspecialty of the physician doing the surgical or medical procedure.
- Hospitals use a spectrum of definitions for operating room time ranging from time between incision and closure to time between administration of anaesthesia and exit from the operating room. Although efforts were made to impose a consistent start and

end definition for operating room time, data within the patient records often were contradictory, making it impossible for coders to determine start and end times.

- There was no consensus regarding what constitutes an operating room and how to define operative procedures. Should invasive diagnostic procedures be included? Should administration of anaesthesia be required for designation as an operative procedure? The latter offered additional difficulties as coding of anaesthesia is optional on the CIHI abstract.
- Hospitals were not consistent in their designation of patients who had been in same-day surgery during the past week or month and then were admitted as inpatients. Most hospitals classified these patients as new admissions but others coded them as readmissions.
- Hospitals also disagreed among themselves, and with the Ministry of Health, regarding what should be considered legitimate same-day surgery procedures.

These data definition problems can result either in large differences in reported events among hospitals when differences actually are minor, or in large amounts of missing data making comparisons impossible. Standardizing data collection would be a major step towards improving the reliability of the data.

Reliability of the three indicators that required the identification of unplanned events were of particular concern to respondents. They questioned the coders' ability to accurately identify unplanned hospital readmission, return to the operating room, and inpatient admission from same-day surgery based on the medical records. Indeed the ability to distinguish between planned and unplanned events is a difficult task. Many of these events may be unplanned but not unexpected given the case history. We developed a detailed algorithm for the coding of these events and also risk-adjusted using the morbidity classification. We found that the proportion of unplanned events increased with the severity of the morbidity classification.

Twenty-two percent of the respondents who did not use the indicator reports were not sure how to use the information, while 40% did not have time to use the information. This suggests that strategies must be developed to facilitate the interpretation and use of performance measures such as these clinical outcome indicators. Difficulty in applying the indicator information may be related to the fact that three of the indicators—unplanned hospital readmission, unplanned return to the operating room, and unplanned inpatient admission from the same-day surgery—were generic rather than diagnosis- or procedure-specific. Although the rates for these three indicators were aggregated by morbidity classification in the comparative report and by morbidity classification and physician specialty in the hospital-specific report, rates for specific diagnoses or procedures might have assisted the recipients of the reports in identifying areas for in-depth monitoring. The rates for caesarean section were by far the most specific. Rates were reported for primary and repeat caesarean section; for vaginal birth following a previous caesarean section, and for repeat caesarean section with and without an attempted vaginal birth. Comments from respondents suggest that the majority of policy and practice changes were associated with the caesarean section indicator information which allowed the identification of specific areas for further investigation. As well, a larger proportion of respondents wanted data collection and exchange to continue for the caesarean section indicators than for the other four indicators. Recent studies have noted a preference for diagnosis-specific and procedure-specific indicators such as those collected in medical audits (Iezzoni, 1994; Davies et al, 1994). The data collection demands for diagnosis- and procedure-specific indicators usually are greater than for generic indicators. However, Palmer (1996) notes that

> clinical performance measurement can be made more affordable by deriving measures from widely used databases, developing and disseminating well-specified measure sets, reusing measure sets to monitor time trends, sampling cases when cost per case is high, and using smaller sample sizes for monitoring performance repeatedly.

Research on innovation diffusion provides a framework for understanding the dissemination and application of new information such as that contained in the indicator reports (Sechrest et al, 1994). A number of strategies have been tested to support the application of research (e.g. clinical guidelines). Strategies include mailed feedback such as that used in this study, academic detailing, working with an opinion leader or educational influential (Lomas and colleagues, 1991, 1988). The literature suggests that greater interaction between the providers of the information and the potential users presents ongoing opportunities for questions, discussion of concerns, and collaborative action that can enhance information use (Jordan et al, 1995).

Finally, two other issues affecting indicator use were identified: the timeliness of the reports and the extent of dissemination. Responses to open-ended questions mentioned that the reports were not timely in that they presented data that was several months old. There was a wide variation among the hospitals in the amount of time taken to submit monthly inpatient discharge data to the CIHI and to complete the corrections for each month of data. The overall time frame for a quarter of inpatient discharge data to reach the research team for analysis and report generation was approximately five months. As the reporting requirements for same-day surgery discharge data are not the same as for inpatient data, the turnaround time for inpatient admission from same-day surgery was more than five months. The research team took an additional six weeks to analyse the data and prepare the reports. Thus, the bulk of the delay occurred during data collection and correction activities.

The use of a central liaison person in each hospital was not an effective dissemination technique. A preferable method would have been to send a copy of the indicator reports to each of the individuals consulted at the beginning of the study regarding the relevance and feasibility of various indicators. This likely would have led to much wider dissemination within each hospital.

In summary, constant interaction with the hospitals is required from the selection of the indicators to be monitored through data collection, report dissemination, and application of indicator information. Concerns about data reliability, comparability, and timeliness suggest that researchers and hospitals should form partnerships to improve data quality and promote clinical practice improvement (Backer, 1995; Davies et al, 1994). Hospitals will need to take a more active role in improving data reliability and timeliness, while researchers need to assume greater responsibility for ensuring indicator validity and for developing effective strategies for disseminating, presenting, and facilitating the use of performance indicators.

8.6 REFERENCES

Backer, T. E. (1995) Integrating behavioral and systems strategies to change clinical practice. *Journal of Quality Improvement*, **21**(7), 351–3.

Bernstein, S. J. & Hilborne, L. H. (1993) Clinical indicators: the road to quality of care? *Journal of Quality Improvement*, **19**(11), 501–9.

Charlson, M. E., Pompei, P., Ales, K. L. & Mackenzie, C. R. (1987) A new method of classifying prognostic comorbidity in longitudinal studies: development and validation. *Journal of Chronic Disease*, **40**(5), 373–83.

Davies, A. R., Thomas Doyle, M. A., Lansky, D., Rutt, W., Orsoltis Stevic, M. & Doyle, J. B. (1994) Outcome assessment in clinical settings: a consensus statement on principles and best practices in project management. *Journal of Quality Improvement*, **20**(1), 6–16.

Donabedian, A. (1980) *The Definition of Quality and Approaches to Its Assessment*. Ann Arbor: Health Administration Press.

Iezzoni, L. I. (ed.) (1994) *Risk Adjustment for Measuring Health Care Outcomes*. Ann Arbor: Health Administration Press.

Jordan, H. S., Straus, J. H. & Bailit, M. H. (1995) Reporting and using health plan performance information in Massachusetts. *Journal of Quality Improvement*, **21**(4), 167–77.

Lohr, K. N. (1988) Outcome measurement: concepts and questions. *Inquiry*, **25**, 37–50.

Lomas, J., Enkin, M., Anderson, G. M. et al (1991) Opinion leaders versus audit and feedback to implement practice guidelines: delivery after previous cesarian section. *Journal of the American Medical Association*, **265**, 2202–7.

Lomas, J. & Haynes, R. B. (1988) A taxonomy and critical review of tested strategies for the application of clinical practice recommendations: from 'official' to 'individual' clinical policy. *American Journal of Preventive Medicine*, **4**(suppl.), 77–94.

O'Leary, D. S. (1993) The measurement mandate: report card day is coming. *Journal of Quality Improvement*, **19**(11), 487–91.

Palmer, R. H. (1996) Measuring clinical performance to provide information for quality improvement. *Quality Management in Health Care*, **4**(2), 1–6.

Reinertsen, J. L. (1993) Outcomes management and continuous quality improvement: the compass and the rudder. *Quality Review Bulletin*, **19**, 5–7.

Sechrest, L., Backer, T. E., Rogers, E. M., Campbell, T. R. & Grady, M. L. (eds) (1994) *Effective Dissemination of Clinical and Health Information*. Rockville, MD: US Department of Health and Human Services.

CHAPTER 9

The Way Forward: Improving the Improvement Process

9.1 CHAPTER SUMMARY

This chapter starts by using the earlier chapters to justify the need for a systematic approach to improving patient care. It outlines a structured approach that seeks to classify clinical audit problems in terms of their information requirements. Once the problem has been classified then the procedure will define the required data and analysis techniques.

Through the establishment of clear aims and objectives a structured approach can greatly simplify the design process. By classifying the objectives in terms of the data associated with them, the structured approach can determine both data and analysis requirements at the start of the audit process, thus ensuring that correct and sufficient data are gathered. The chapter outlines the method and provides suitable documentation. This is a very practical chapter.

It concludes with a summary of benefits to be expected from using the method.

9.2 THE NEED FOR A SYSTEMATIC APPROACH

The need for a more systematic approach to improving patient care has been seen in earlier chapters. Approaches such as clinical audit are being applied in an incomplete manner. Experience from other places such as Toronto suggests an unwillingness to change working practices.

A systematic and structured approach can only provide a basis for improvement. Implementation of better patient care ultimately rests with the dedication and professionalism of the individual healthcare workers and managers. However, without proper tools, the most dedicated worker cannot do a proper job.

The approach outlined is intended to address the following issues:

- to ensure that improvement effort is focused effectively
- to ensure that clear goals are set
- to ensure that all required data are collected
- to ensure that data analysis is accurate and complete
- to ensure that findings are translated into better practice
- to ensure that improvement is an ongoing process.

There is an emphasis on the need for improvement rather than the need to measure current performance. Although the approach may be applied within a clinical audit context, this is not a requirement. The process seeks to achieve the stated aim of audit—i.e. to improve patient care—rather than to reinforce the limitations of current practice where too often audit does not proceed beyond data collection and analysis and the opportunity to feed back findings into practice is lost.

The method is based upon two underlying approaches:

- the structured approach to problem solving
- the cycle, found in clinical audit and process improvement.

The Structured Approach to Problem Solving

The structured approach to problem solving is derived from engineering. It is hierarchical or tree-like in nature and is based upon breaking down a task into smaller components.

Consider the problem of washing up. In many households this is a very unstructured process. However, it is perfectly possible to view washing up as a structured process. First we must establish what it is we are trying to achieve. This is our aim:

Aim. 'The aim of washing up is to clean the dishes and utensils used in a meal as effectively and efficiently as possible.'

This can then be expressed as a set of objectives which if carried out will enable us to achieve our overall aim. The objectives in our washing up example are summarized in Table 9.1.

Each objective must then be fulfilled if the overall aim is to be achieved. This leads to each objective defining a task. If each task is completed successfully, then each objective will be realized and the overall aim will have been achieved.

This approach is at the heart of any quality management system, where the overall task is modelled as a series of processes. In this way the overall task is represented in terms of a series of sub-tasks. The quality management system provides a systematic way of carrying out each sub-task and dealing with any departures from the approved system.

However, such systems are often poor at correcting errors and improving the methods for carrying out tasks. Therefore, the structured approach must be combined with a mechanism for actually improving care where an investigation reveals shortcomings. This is achieved by combining a structured approach with an improvement cycle.

The Improvement Cycle

The cycle is at the heart of classical process improvement and clinical procedures. However, we have seen evidence that it is not

Table 9.1 Objectives for washing up

(1)	To sort washing up into categories
(2)	To clean surfaces
(3)	To rinse dishes
(4)	To wash glasses
(5)	To wash cutlery
(6)	To wash crockery
(7)	To wash pots and pans
(8)	To dry glasses, dry cutlery, dry crockery, dry pots and pans
(9)	To put away dishes
(10)	To clean up sink area and bowl

being completed in the case of many clinical audits. The seven-stage process shown in Fig. 9.1 combines a structured approach to design and analysis with the vital stages of the implementation of change and subsequent evaluation.

This can be seen as an approach to the implementation of existing ideas rather than another new method. Each stage will now be examined in detail, followed by a description of a practical paper-based method. A computer-based tool is currently under development.

9.3   DISCUSSION OF EACH STAGE OF THE PROCESS

Stage 1: Design of Investigation

The design of the investigation is crucial. The establishment of clear aims and objectives will facilitate each following stage. We

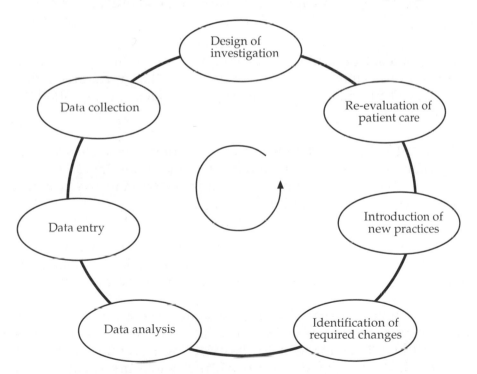

Figure 9.1   Seven-stage model of improving patient care

shall use a model investigation to illustrate the application of the approach, supported by other examples as necessary.

In the model investigation, the quality of care within an infertility clinic has been called into question by an external report into the quality of care provided nationwide. The report suggests that a particular clinical procedure (a laparoscopy and dye test) should be carried out only by senior clinicians. Further it suggests that pathology investigations are often carried out in a limited manner only. The study is set up to investigate the quality of care provided in a particular hospital and to bring it into line with the report's recommendations.

The overall design process is shown in Fig. 9.2. The first stage is to establish a clear aim. The statement of aim should be a single statement, and all that follows should flow from it. For our example, the aim may be stated as:

Aim. To improve the quality of care provided to patients undergoing a laparoscopy and dye test in the infertility clinic.

The statement of aim may be refined by a statement of scope. The statement of scope defines the limits of the investigation. in terms of the patient sample to be used and the procedures under scrutiny. Thus, in our case the scope is defined in the following manner:

Scope. The investigation is concerned with patients attending the Infertility Clinic between January 1st and June 1st, 1992. The procedures under scrutiny are the laparoscopy and dye test and associated admissions and pathology procedures.

Once the aim and scope are determined then the objectives may be established. An objective is a statement of how a particular factor is to be investigated to contribute to the overall aim of the study.

In the first instance, the objectives are used to determine the information requirements of the study. However, as improvements can only be made on the basis of findings from information gathered, they do in practice drive the whole investigation. For the model investigation, the following objectives were established:

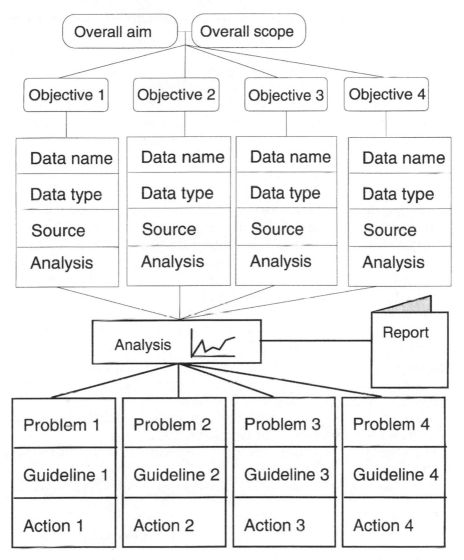

Figure 9.2 Graphical representation of the design phase

(1) To investigate the status of the operator
(2) To investigate delays between appointments and requests for tests
(3) To investigate delays between requests and the tests themselves

(4)   To investigate the thoroughness of pathological investigation in such cases.

Stage 2: Data Collection

In order to meet the first objective, it is necessary to record the status of the doctor, either as consultant (C), or registrar (R), or senior house officer (S). This leads to the set of data and analysis requirements summarized in Table 9.2.

In order to meet Objectives 2 and 3, it is necessary to collect two pieces of data for each patient, the date of a request for an appointment and the date of the actual appointment. A piece of data is stored in a database within a *field*. Each field has a predefined type. The field types available include freeform, alpha-numeric, numeric (integer or real) and dates. In this case, the required fields are dates and may be gathered from patient records (see Table 9.3).

The analysis required is to establish the number of days between the two dates (d) and to consider performance in terms of d. To define the distribution of d, the mean value of d and the dispersion measured as the *standard deviation* are required. A histogram of the distribution may also prove helpful.

Objective 4 may be considered by collecting data on which specific tests were carried out (see Table 9.4).

Thus the data sheet defined for the investigation would include the fields shown in Table 9.5.

It is also necessary to decide whether any subsidiary data are

Table 9.2   Requirements associated with Objective 1

Data required:	Doctor status
Data fields:	Alphanumeric: 'C', 'R', 'S'
Data source:	Patient or clinic records
Analysis:	% of patients seen by a consultant
	% of patients seen by a registrar
	% of patients seen by an SHO
	Pie chart to illustrate factors

Table 9.3 Requirements associated with Objective 2

Data required:	Date requested, Date of appointment
Data fields:	[Date1], [Date2]
Data source:	Patient records
Analysis:	$d := [Date2] - [Date1]$
	$\bar{d}, \sigma_d$
	Histogram of d

Note: $\bar{d}$ is the mean waiting time in days, and σ_d is the standard deviation of the waiting time

Table 9.4 Requirements associated with Objective 4

Data required:	Pathology test carried out
Data fields:	[Yes/No]
Data source:	Patient records
Analysis:	% of patients having test

required to break down the groups further. For example, the clinic is run by four consultant firms and analysis of practice should distinguish between these.

Sources of Data

The data may be collected from a variety of sources. These may be considered under three broad headings:

- historical paper-based patient records
- computer-based patient records
- 'live' patient survey.

Specific sources are given in Table 9.6.

Historical data are often the easiest to deal with, having already been collected. The data may even exist in electronic form. The drawbacks are that the data may not have been collected in the

Table 9.5 Quality of care associated with laparoscopy and dye test: data sheet

Field name	Field type	Explanatory notes
Patient no.	[nnn]	Three-digit code to identify patients
Consultant firm	[n]	Four consultant firms operate the clinic; identified by single digit 1–4
Operator ⟨A⟩	[A]	Single letter: C, R or S identifies operator as consultant, registrar or senior house officer
Appointment date	[dd/mm/yy]	Date of initial consultation
Date test requested	[dd/mm/yy]	Date test requested
Test date	[dd/mm/yy]	Date test carried out
Endometriosis	[Yes/No]	Test for endometriosis carried out?
PID	[Yes/No]	Test for PID carried out?
Adhesions	[Yes/No]	Test for adhesions carried out?
Semen analysis	[Yes/No]	Semen analysis carried out?
Culture	[Yes/No]	Cultured?
MAR	[Yes/No]	MAR performed?
Endocrine profile	[Yes/No]	Endocrine profile carried out?
Post-coital test	[Yes/No]	Post-coital test carried out?

form that you need. More seriously, it is not always easy to verify accuracy. Audits based upon historical data should carry a caveat to the effect that the quality of the results is subject to factors beyond the control of the audit team.

It is often useful to supplement historical data with data gathered specifically for the investigation, since the requirements may not always mirror the clinicians' information needs. However, since the process is designed to improve patient care, an intrusive data gathering process may be counterproductive. Any demands upon staff to collect extra data may lead to less time with patients and fewer patients seen.

Table 9.6 Sources of data (after Hunt and Legg, 1994)

Source type	Sources	Examples
Historical (paper)	Registers	Cancer registry, diagnostic index, child health registers
	Departmental records	Appointment books, pharmacy, theatre books
	Professional notes	District nursing notes, ward kardex
Historical (computer)	Computer-based	Korner data, PAS, case mix system
'Live' data	Surveys	Postal questionnaire, questionnaire at clinic, patient interviews

Surveys of patients may be the only way to gather data on patients' perceptions of care. If quality of care is to be taken seriously, then patients' perceptions are crucial. For example, a patient may be happier waiting an extra ten minutes to see a doctor if that results in an extra ten minutes in the consultation.

Patient questionnaires must be carried out with great care if a true reflection of patient views is to be obtained. A full treatment of questionnaire design and other related issues such as sampling is beyond the scope of this book. The interested reader is referred to specialist texts such as Abramson (1984). However, the following questions should be considered:

- How are the questionnaires to reach the patients?
- How will you ensure that the sample of patients who reply is representative of the whole?
- How can you maximize the response rate to gain a significant result?
- How do you ensure that the questionnaire actually asks what you want it to, and does not bias the outcome by its construction?

Once the data collection has been designed, the data must be actually collected and entered into a database, usually computer-based.

Stage 3: Data Entry

The task of data entry is dull but crucial. Unless the data exist in a compatible electronic form, most investigations will require manual data entry. Two types of data entry errors can arise:

(a) *Impossible values*. These errors arise when the data entered cannot be a valid response. Specifying the field type will provide elementary protection against the wrong type of data being entered. More specific protection such as limiting valid responses to the operator field—in our example to C, R or S must be specified.
(b) *Incorrect but possible values*. These errors are much more difficult to prevent. They arise when the value entered is incorrect but could be a possible answer. Usually, these errors are reduced by carrying out the data entry process twice. If two independent operators enter the same data with reasonable accuracy, the chance of them putting in the same random error is very small. Therefore, discrepancies between the two data sets indicate errors in one set or other.

The computer software chosen to carry out data entry and analysis is a matter of taste and availability. The author favours a piece of software produced by the World Health Organization and the Centers for Disease Control and Prevention, known as Epi Info (Dean et al, 1995). This software is available free of charge and provides excellent data entry and analysis features. It does, however, look rather old fashioned. Use of Epi Info in investigations is covered in detail in Gillies (1995). Alternatively, the use of a commercial package such as Excel is covered in Gillies and Baugh (1994). The approach is not, however, software dependent.

Stage 4: Data Analysis

The analysis of data can appear to be a very complex business. With the availability of PCs, there is a temptation to believe that it is necessary to provide complex statistical justifications for all findings because the means are there. However, there are some very good reasons why such complicated analysis is often not required:

(1) The data do not justify it.
(2) The problem doesn't need it.
(3) It wouldn't tell your target audience anything anyway.
(4) Data analysis is a means to an end: the goal is the improvement of patient care.

First consider the question of the data. There are two issues, quality and quantity. Any study is dependent upon the data on which it is based. Many studies are based upon small sample sizes. Where the sample size is small, the number of statistically valid conclusions that may be drawn is relatively small.

Data analysis is once again determined by the objectives. Objectives may be classified according to three characteristics of the data associated with them:

- type (simple, multiple or derived)
- range (single, binary or multiple)
- dimensions (one-dimensional, two-dimensional etc.).

If these three characteristics are identified for each objective then this will enable us to define all the information we need to design the analysis of our data.

Data Types

Simple data arise where the factor to be investigated may be found directly. For example if our objective states that we wish to investigate the status of a doctor seeing a patient in a clinic, then the status of the doctor is directly identifiable and therefore is simple.

Multiple data arise where the factor to be investigated is directly identifiable but is made up of several individual pieces of data. For example in our infertility study, one of the objectives is to investigate the thoroughness of pathological investigation. This factor is represented by three separate pieces of data each indicating whether a specific test has been carried out.

Derived data arise where the factor to be investigated must be calculated from the data collected. For example, if our objective is to investigate the time between referral and consultation, the actual data required are derived from two other pieces of data, the date of referral and the date of consultation.

Data Range

Single range data consist of a single piece of information. Examples of data of this type are the age, sex and weight of the patient. Dates are a common form of single range data, usually found in an objective where the required data are derived from several pieces of single range data.

Binary range data arise where the data are either positive or negative. For example, has a specific test been carried out? Once again this form of data is most commonly found in derived or multiple data type objectives, e.g. the thoroughness of pathological investigation which is an example of a multiple type binary range objective.

Multiple range data arise where the data have three or more possible values. Examples seen thus far include the status of an operating doctor, which has three possible values—consultant, registrar, or senior house officer—and the satisfaction of patients, which has five possible values between very satisfied and very dissatisfied.

Data Dimensions

One-dimensional data arise where the objective investigates the distribution of data across the whole population at once. Thus, the status of a doctor is one-dimensional.

Two-dimensional data arise where the investigation breaks down the distribution of data according to the distribution of a second factor. Thus if we investigate the status of a doctor broken down by consulting firm we obtain two-dimensional data.

Multiple-dimensional data analysis is possible, but with simple analysis tools such as Epi Info, it is only possible to achieve this by representing multi-dimensional analysis by a series of two-dimensional analyses.

The foregoing classification leads to 18 possible objective types, summarized in Table 9.7. Of these, 14 are found in practice.

Applying the Principles to One-Dimensional Analysis

The simplest type of objective has a simple data type and a single data range—e.g. to investigate the bodyweight of patients. The analysis required in this case is to show the distribution of

Table 9.7 Eighteen objective types (14 found in practice)

Type	Range	Dimensions	Example objective
Simple	Single	One	Weight distribution of patients
Multiple	Single	One	Blood pressure distribution of patients
Derived	Single	One	Waiting time for patients
Simple	Binary	One	Sex distribution of patients
Multiple	Binary	One	Presence of symptoms amongst patients
Derived	Binary	One	Not generally found in practice
Simple	Multiple	One	Satisfaction of patients
Multiple	Multiple	One	Satisfaction of patients across a number of factors
Derived	Multiple	One	Not generally found in practice
Simple	Single	Two	Weight distributions of patients grouped by consultant
Multiple	Single	Two	Blood pressure distributions of patients grouped by consultant
Derived	Single	Two	Waiting times for patients grouped by consultant
Simple	Binary	Two	Sex distributions of patients grouped by consultant
Multiple	Binary	Two	Presence of symptoms amongst patients grouped by consultant
Derived	Binary	Two	Not generally found in practice
Simple	Multiple	Two	Satisfaction of patients grouped by consultant
Multiple	Multiple	Two	Satisfaction of patients across a number of factors grouped by consultant
Derived	Multiple	Two	Not generally found in practice

bodyweight within the population under consideration. The distribution may be defined by the mean bodyweight, the standard deviation and by a histogram of the data. In this case where the data have a single range, the data must be grouped for the histogram.

If the data type is multiple, such as in the case of blood pressure, then the data sets are treated separately. In this case, the data required are a number for the diastolic blood pressure and one for the systolic pressure. The means and standard deviations should be calculated separately and the histograms plotted as two sets of grouped data. Thus this type of data would produce the following results:

- mean diastolic blood pressure
- mean systolic blood pressure
- standard deviation in the diastolic blood pressure
- standard deviation in the systolic blood pressure
- histogram of diastolic blood pressure distribution
- histogram of systolic blood pressure distribution.

With derived data, the final data are derived before analysis. Thus, in the case of the time between referral and appointment required by Objective 2 of our earlier example, the time is first calculated, then treated as a simple data case.

An objective requiring data with a binary range such as the sex distribution of a patient population is somewhat simpler. Provided the data are one-dimensional, then the data may be simply analysed as a percentage and supported by a pie chart if graphical representation is required.

Multiple binary data are treated similarly, except that for graphical representation the percentages are best collated as a bar chart. Consider, for example, the data associated with Objective 4 in our earlier example (to investigate the thoroughness of pathological investigation). The data associated with this objective are stored as binary variables:

Endometriosis	[Yes/No]	Culture	[Yes/No]
PID	[Yes/No]	MAR	[Yes/No]
Adhesions	[Yes/No]	Endocrine profile	[Yes/No]
Semen analysis	[Yes/No]	Post-coital test	[Yes/No]

Where the data have a multiple range but are defined by a simple variable, then the analysis techniques required are the mean, the standard deviation and a histogram. This analysis was considered when the satisfaction measures were discussed earlier.

More complicated is the situation where the data required are collected as a set of variables, each with a multiple range. In general, these are best treated as a group of simple variables, but the graphs may be collated for comparison purposes. We might, for example, wish to combine patient satisfaction measures covering a number of issues into an overall measure of satisfaction. Arithmetic combination will reduce the quality of the data available, but graphical comparison of each factor may be helpful, as shown in Fig. 9.3.

Results such as those illustrated would indicate that there was dissatisfaction with the issue 1, but not with issue 2. Numerical combination would lose the discrimination between factors.

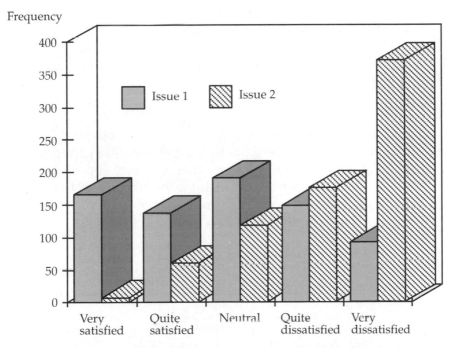

Figure 9.3 Collated graph derived from multiple binary data

Applying the Principles to Two-Dimensional Analysis

All the cases thus far have been concerned with one-dimensional analysis. Now we shall consider each case again, this time breaking down the data set by another factor.

The simplest case of two-dimensional analysis is where the data type is simple and the data range is single. Thus we can revisit our weight distribution example above and this time break it down according to consultant. The analysis of weight broken down by consultant is shown in Table 9.8. We now treat each column as a separate set of data, but otherwise analyse as before, producing a mean and standard deviation for each set of figures.

If comparison is required then a grouped three-dimensional histogram may be provided. However, care is required if clarity is not to be sacrificed. If we simply plot the equivalent histogram to that produced earlier, the result is attractive but unclear. However, it may be better to present each graph separately but aligned vertically to allow for comparison. It is an increasing problem that modern computer software is capable of producing graphs that, while stunning visually, do not communicate the required message, which is to highlight areas in need of improvement.

Similar considerations apply to cases where the data types are multiple, as in the blood pressure example, or derived as in the waiting time example. In each case the data may be divided according to a second variable, such as consultant, and then evaluated.

Where the data are simple, but have a binary range, (such as the sex of the patients), and we wish to present the data grouped by a further variable in a graphical form, then we may choose between multiple pie charts or a grouped histogram—according to whether we wish to emphasize comparison between patient groups or within them. The multiple pie chart option emphasizes the intra-

Table 9.8   Sample bodyweight: analysis results

Consultant	Brown	Jones	Smith
Mean (kg)	71.88	69.35	68.93
Standard deviation (kg)	7.75	10.24	10.42

group relationships, whilst the histogram invites comparison between groups.

Where the data range is multiple rather than binary, we may now start to look for relationships between the data types. For example, if we consider the case of looking at patient satisfaction ratings grouped by consultant, we can investigate whether there is a relationship between the two. However, at this stage we shall consider the simpler case where the data type is simple in type but multiple in range, because the approach to be adopted is similar in both cases. Consider the sample data shown in Table 9.9.

A simplistic view such as assigning a score to each rating and calculating a mean score reveals little. This could be enhanced by a graph of the relative distribution. However, it is worth considering whether this adds to our understanding of the factor under consideration.

A better approach uses a *chi-squared test* to evaluate the probability of a link between patient satisfaction and the consultant concerned. A chi-squared analysis carried out using Excel is shown in Fig. 9.4.

A very low *p*-value indicates that there is a strong relationship between patients' views and the doctor concerned. A similar approach may be used to compare relationships between different factors where the data type is multiple.

Table 9.10 attempts to summarize the analysis options. However, if you're put off by a lot of Greek letters, then move on swiftly and you will not be greatly disadvantaged!

Table 9.9　Sample satisfaction data by consultant

Rating	Rating score	Consultant		
		Brown	Green	White
Very satisfied	+2	45	34	56
Quite satisfied	+1	34	53	12
No strong feelings	0	21	23	2
Quite dissatisfied	−1	6	3	18
Very dissatisfied	−2	0	1	5
Mean score		1.11	1.02	1.03

	A	B	C	D	E
1	Actual	Brown	Green	White	
2	Very satisfied	45	34	56	135
3	Quite satisfied	34	53	12	99
4	No strong feelings	21	23	2	46
5	Quite dissatisfied	6	3	18	27
6	Very dissatisfied	0	1	5	6
7		106	114	93	313
8	Expected	Brown	Green	White	
9	Very satisfied	45.71885	49.16933	40.11182	135
10	Quite satisfied	33.52716	36.05751	29.41534	99
11	No strong feelings	15.57827	16.75399	13.66773	46
12	Quite dissatisfied	9.14377	9.833866	8.022364	27
13	Very dissatisfied	2.031949	2.185304	1.782748	6
14		106	114	93	313
15					
16	p-value	4.57E-12			

Figure 9.4   Chi-squared analysis using Excel

Stage 5: Identification of Required Changes

If the cycle is viewed as two halves, the first concerned with evaluation, the second with improvement, then we are now entering the stages concerned directly with improvement.

Identification of changes is carried out for each objective of the study. The process may be illustrated as a flow chart (see Fig. 9.5).

Stage 6: Introduction of New Practices

Change is rarely popular. In healthcare where professionalism is highly prized and rightly so, then change must be carefully managed. Oakland (1989) points out that changes must be 'sold' to staff, and the benefits of better practice emphasized, including

- greater job satisfaction
- less time wasted on pointless activity
- greater pride in work.

Table 9.10 Summary of analysis techniques required by each objective type

Type	Range	Dimensions	Analysis techniques
Simple	Single	One	x/n, σ_x; histogram (x_{grp})
Multiple	Single	One	x_i/n, σx_i, $\Sigma x_j/n$, σx_j, …; histogram (x_{i-grp}, x_{j-grp}, …)
Derived	Single	One	$z = f(x)$, $\Sigma z/n$, σ_z; histogram (z)
Simple	Binary	One	$\%x_1$, $\%x_2$; pie ($\%x_1$, $\%x_2$)
Multiple	Binary	One	$\%x_{i=1}$, $\%x_{j=1}$, $\%x_{k=1}$; histogram ($\%x_{i=1}$, $\%x_{j=1}$, $\%x_{k=1}$)
Simple	Multiple	One	x/n, σ_x; histogram (x)
Multiple	Multiple	One	x_i/n, σx_i, $\Sigma x_j/n$, σx_j, …; histogram ($x_i, x_j, \ldots$)
Simple	Single	Two	(x, y); $\Sigma y/n$; σ_y; histogram (y)
Multiple	Single	Two	(x, y); $\Sigma y/n$; σ_y; histogram (y)
Derived	Single	Two	$z = f(x)$, (z, y): $\Sigma y/n$, σ_y; histogram (y)
Simple	Binary	Two	Crosstab (x, y); pie (x) for each y or grouped histogram (x, y)
Multiple	Binary	Two	Crosstab (x, y); pie (x) for each y or grouped histogram (x, y)
Simple	Multiple	Two	Crosstab (x, y); $P(\chi^2)$
Multiple	Multiple	Two	Crosstab (x, y); $P(\chi^2)$

In practice, dedication and professionalism should help the introduction of new practices where a clear benefit to patients can be seen.

One of the defining characteristics of clinical audit is local ownership and control. This can greatly enhance the likelihood of the acceptance of change, and is one of the key advantages of local clinical audits over imposed 'top-down' quality assurance procedures.

One disadvantage of local audits is the problem of wider dissemination and change. This is a two-fold problem:

(a) *Dissemination of findings to a wider audience.* This is a simple communication problem. As an example, in the Oxford and Four Counties region, only about 1–2% of audits are published in the *Auditorium* journal (see Chapter 6).

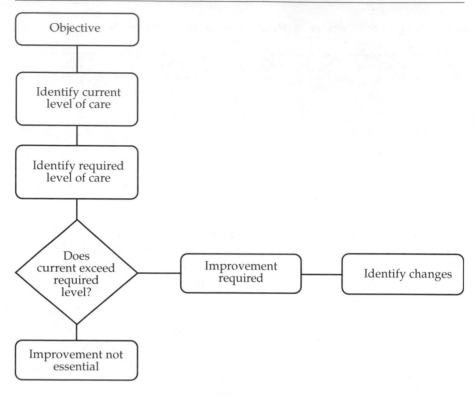

Figure 9.5   Process of identifying problem areas

(b) *Application of change in a different environment.* Many of the findings of clinical audit investigations will be relevant to other locations. However, these sites no longer have local ownership of the findings and may resist change on the grounds of 'not invented here'.

Stage 7: Re-evaluation of Patient Care

Only 47% of the audits covered by the study described in Chapter 6 showed a commitment to re-audit and complete the cycle. For the reasons described in Chapter 6, the global figure is likely to be lower.

The re-audit step must be designed into the overall audit process. A commitment to reconsider levels of care under each objective must be made at the design stage. The time to re-audit will depend upon:

- the type of problem under scrutiny (patient, clinical, resource)
- the level of activity
- the degree of change
- the time for change actually to be introduced.

A balance needs to be struck between the need to provide information about the benefits derived from change in practice and the time for change to take effect. Further, too frequent re-audits may distract resources away from the primary task of patient care.

9.4   PRACTICAL IMPLEMENTATION OF THE METHOD

The approach may be implemented in a seven-stage model as shown in Fig. 9.6. At the design stage, eight questions need to be considered:

(1)   What is the overall aim of the audit?
(2)   What objectives must be set to meet this aim?
(3)   What data must be collected to ensure that each objective is realized?
(4)   How will the data be collected?
(5)   How will the data be analysed?
(6)   What changes in practice are required?
(7)   How will the changes be implemented?
(8)   How will be the effect of the change be evaluated?

If these eight questions are answered effectively the design and implementation should proceed smoothly. In order to ensure that these questions are investigated in a systematic manner, the author has developed a *paper-based design method*. A computer-based tool is currently under development. The paper forms are distributed as a Word for Windows computer disk. This allows the user to add extra detail where required.

Section 1 deals with aims and objectives. These have been

described earlier in this chapter. Up to five objectives are provided for on the standard form.

In Section 2, the data needed to meet the requirements of each objective are entered on the form. Up to three fields are permitted on the standard form. Each is defined by name, type and size where required. Names should be up to 10 characters long to allow direct translation into Epi field names. Data types should be one of:

- Alphanumeric: text and numbers
- Numeric: numbers
- Date: date format
- Yes/No: allows Yes or No or Don't Know as a response.

The data size is applicable only to alphanumeric or numeric fields. It indicates the length of the string in the case of an alphanumeric field or the number of digits in the case of a numeric variable. If there is a figure after the decimal point it indicates the number of decimal places in a real number.

Section 3 is concerned with the classification of the data associated with each objective. The objectives may be classified according to the type of data associated with them. Thus this table has entries for the data type range and dimensions associated with each objective. From these, the analysis technique to be used may be derived. The suggested analysis methods may be determined from Fig. 9.2.

Section 4 is self-explanatory. The results of the analysis may form the basis of the audit report, but this is not the end of the process. The next stage is the identification of required changes.

In Section 5, for each objective, the current performance level is derived from the analysis stage. This may be compared with a target level of performance. Where the current level does not exceed the target performance, changes in procedures must be identified.

For each change identified, the re-audit date must be set. This is the final step in the process, completing the audit cycle.

The approach is illustrated for the model audit investigation in Fig. 9.7.

AUDIT INVESTIGATION: DESIGN FORM

SECTION 1: AIMS AND OBJECTIVES

The aim of the audit study is to _____

_____

_____

The objectives which must be met are:

Objective 1: To _____

_____

Objective 2: To _____

_____

Objective 3: To _____

_____

Objective 4: To _____

_____

Figure 9.6 Paper-based structured method for audit

SECTION 2: DATA REQUIREMENTS			
Objective	Data name	Type/size	Source
1			
2			
3			
4			

Figure 9.6   (*continued*)

SECTION 3: DATA ANALYSIS				
Objective	Data classification			Analysis method
	Type	Range	Dims	
1				
2				
3				
4				

SECTION 4: DISSEMINATION REQUIREMENTS

The dissemination requirements of the study are:
(Tick all appropriate sections subject to available resources)

Interactive analysis   ☐

Automated analysis   ☐

Generated report   ☐

OHP slides   ☐

Further analysis   ☐

Figure 9.6   *(continued)*

SECTION 5: IDENTIFICATION OF PROBLEMS AND REMEDIAL ACTIONS

Objective 1 current level of performance:
Objective 1 target level of performance:
Change implemented ☐   Date for re-audit: _____
Objective 2 current level of performance:
Objective 2 target level of performance:
Change implemented ☐   Date for re-audit: _____
Objective 3 current level of performance:
Objective 3 target level of performance:
Change implemented ☐   Date for re-audit: _____
Objective 4 current level of performance:
Objective 4 target level of performance:
Change implemented ☐   Date for re-audit: _____

Figure 9.6   (*continued*)

AUDIT INVESTIGATION: DESIGN FORM

SECTION 1: AIMS AND OBJECTIVES

The aim of the audit study is to _examine the quality of care provided to patients undergoing a laparoscopy and dye test in the infertility clinic._

The objectives which must be met are:

Objective 1: To _investigate the status of the operator._

Objective 2: To _investigate delays between appointments and requests for tests_

Objective 3: To _investigate delays between requests and the test themselves._

Objective 4: To _investigate the thoroughness of pathological investigation in such cases._

Figure 9.7 Completed design form for the model investigation

SECTION 2: DATA REQUIREMENTS			
Objective	Data name	Type/size	Source
1	Operator	Alphanum (1)	Historical (paper)
	Firm	Number (1)	Historical (paper)
2	Appmt_Date	Date	Historical (paper)
	Reqst_Date	Date	Historical (paper)
3	Test_Date	Date	Historical (paper)
	Endometriosis	YES/NO	Historical (paper)
4	PID	YES/NO	Historical (paper)
	Adhesions	YES/NO	Historical (paper)
	Performed	YES/NO	Historical (paper)
	Culture	YES/NO	Historical (paper)
	MAR	YES/NO	Historical (paper)
	Endocrine	YES/NO	Historical (paper)
	Type	Number (1)	Historical (paper)
	Post-coital	YES/NO	Historical (paper)

Figure 9.7   (*continued*)

SECTION 3: DATA ANALYSIS				
Objective	Data classification			Analysis method
	Type	Range	Dims	
1	S	M	2	Crosstab; Chi-squared test
2	D	S	1	Mean; StanDev; Histogram
3	D	S	1	Mean; StanDev; Histogram
4	M	B	1	Fraction; Histogram

SECTION 4: DISSEMINATION REQUIREMENTS

The dissemination requirements of the study are:
(Tick all appropriate sections subject to available resources)

Interactive analysis   ☑

Automated analysis   ☐

Generated report   ☑

OHP slides   ☐

Further analysis   ☐

Figure 9.7   *(continued)*

SECTION 5: IDENTIFICATION OF PROBLEMS AND REMEDIAL ACTIONS

Objective 1 current level of performance: 69% of test procedures are being carried out by staff other than consultants
Objective 1 target level of performance: 75% of procedures to be carried out by consultants No procedures to be carried out by doctors other than senior registrars or consultants
Change implemented ☑   Date for re-audit: 01/06/1993
Objective 2 current level of performance: Mean waiting time for consultations is 9 months Maximum waiting time is 21 months
Objective 2 target level of performance: No patient to wait more than 6 months for consultations
Change implemented ☑   Date for re-audit: 01/12/1993
Objective 3 current level of performance: Mean waiting time between consultation and test is 6 months Maximum waiting time is 12 months
Objective 3 target level of performance: No patient to wait more than 3 months for consultations
Change implemented ☑   Date for re-audit: 01/12/1993
Objective 4 current level of performance: 31% of patients receiving comprehensive pathology investigation in support of test
Objective 4 target level of performance: Agreed set of tests to be used for all patients or exceptions documented
Change implemented ☑   Date for re-audit: 01/06/1993

Figure 9.7   *(continued)*

9.5   BENEFITS SOUGHT FROM THE STRUCTURED METHOD

In other disciplines, structured methods have facilitated the introduction of systematic procedures. It is hoped that this method will achieve the same result within clinical audit.

In the first instance, it is hoped that the structured approach will deliver what is promised in the Department of Health's original definition of clinical audit:

> The systematic, critical analysis of the quality of medical care, including the procedures used for diagnosis and treatment, the use of resources and the resulting outcome and quality of life for the patient.

Audit carried out using the structured approach should be systematic, it should be analytical, and it should be concerned with the quality of care.

If the structured method is successful in achieving these goals, then it will achieve the greater goal of making a significant contribution to the improvement of patient care.

9.6   REFERENCES

Abramson, J. H. (1984) *Survey Methods in Community Medicine*. Edinburgh: Churchill Livingstone.

Dean, J. A., Dean, A. G., Coulombie, D., Smith, D. C., Brendel, K. A. & Arner, T. G. (1995) *Epi Info Version 6: A Word-Processing, Database and Statistics Program for Epidemiology on Microcomputers*. Atlanta, GE: Centers for Disease Control and Prevention (available from USD Inc., 2075A West Park Place, Stone Mountain, GA 30087, USA; fax +404-469-0681).

Gillies, A. C. (1995) The computerisation of general practice: an IT perspective. *Journal of Information Technology*, **10**(1), 75–85.

Gillies, A. C. & Baugh, P. (1994) *Excel in Health Care*. London: Chapman & Hall.

Hunt, V. & Legg, F. (1994) *Clinical Audit: A Basic Introduction*. Oxford University: Regional Postgraduate Medical Education & Training Office.

Oakland, J. (1989) *Total Quality Management*. London: Heinemann.

CHAPTER 10

Conclusions

10.1 CHAPTER SUMMARY

In this chapter we shall conclude by drawing together the main themes of the book and then outline the challenges for the future.

10.2 PROGRESS TO DATE

The desire to improve patient care is not new. Even in the nineteenth century Florence Nightingale was able to dramatically improve the quality of healthcare provided for patients. Some clinicians have resisted the introduction of techniques such as clinical audit, arguing that it is no more than clinical research carried out by any responsible clinician who has the best interests of the patients at heart. However, formal quality assurance procedures do offer a number of advantages:

- *System*. Without a formal programme of quality assurance, activity tends to be sporadic in nature and patchy in coverage.
- *Formal methods*. Informal activity is often carried out in a less rigorous manner than activity which is part of a formal programme with prescribed methods and specific training programmes in audit methods.
- *Focus*. Clinical research should necessarily be more open-ended than quality assurance activity. Audits should have as their principal aim changing practice and improving patient care.

These benefits are being demonstrated in improvements to patient care, and a formal commitment to clinical audit has now been established as part of clinical culture in the NHS. There remain, however, a significant range of challenges for the future.

10.3   CHALLENGES FOR THE FUTURE

Practitioner Resistance

In spite of widespread quality assurance activity amongst clinicians, it is unclear how many practitioners actually undertake such activities out of conviction rather than under coercion. Reasons for resistance vocalized to the author include:

- the view that quality assurance is part of management in a culture where management is seen as an imposition
- the view that quality assurance is used to question professional judgement and integrity
- the fear that it may be demonstrated that current practice is inadequate and therefore by extension so is the practitioner
- the view that quality assurance is simply about saving money rather than improving the quality of patient care.

As with many opinions, these all have an element of truth about them. Indeed, some results will demonstrate how care may be improved and money saved, such as by reducing unnecessary intrusive surgical procedures. Others may well point to problems which can be only be addressed by spending more resources. It is important for staff morale that where money is saved in one area, some evidence of it being used to improve care in another area may be seen.

However, each of the arguments cited above may be countered:

- The vast majority of clinical audit studies are initiated or led by practitioners. Even the diehard opponents argue that quality assurance is part of normal professional activity, so this is an argument about approach, not principle.
- In a clinician-led audit study, the questioning of existing practice is peer-led. Professional practice must evolve or skills

and expertise will become outmoded and obsolete. The professional who should be more worried is the one who has been working the same way without questioning for the last thirty years or so.

- Once again, inadequacy is more likely demonstrated by a refusal to change rather than by the discovery that current practice can be improved. Process improvement is based upon the premise that all practice can be improved. This may be perceived more positively than approaches based upon error elimination.
- All public healthcare environments live with a finite resource allocation. Therefore, saving money in one procedure should allow more provision elsewhere. Since one of the aspects of healthcare is how much can be delivered within a finite budget, then productivity and quality are more closely linked than in manufacturing, for example.

Methods

In spite of a considerable investment in training and education, many studies still fail to use proper methods for clinical audit and other quality assurance activities. This is demonstrated by the fact that in the study cited in Chapter 6, and other similar studies, change in practice is only achieved in less than 50% of cases and the level of re-audit activity is even lower.

Through the structured method outlined in the previous chapter, and through the provision of a tool associated with it, it is hoped to both improve practice and make good practice easier to implement.

Implementing Change

Perhaps the biggest challenge is actually implementing the changes highlighted by the audit investigation. Unless the practitioners involved feel that they have ownership over the changes, then they will almost certainly resist them as imposed from above. Whereas in a hierarchical organization, imposed change may be feasible, change by consensus is the only realistic approach within a professional environment.

Therefore it is vital that clinicians be involved in every stage of the quality assurance process. After that, it is about actively trying to minimize the fears detailed above, and avoiding actions which reinforce prejudice.

10.4   FINAL THOUGHTS

Throughout this book it has been emphasized that there are many different views of quality. It has also been suggested that, although there are many different techniques, there are two broad approaches to quality management—fitness for purpose or conformance to predetermined levels of performance.

These give rise to two types of techniques, clinical audit based upon the audit cycle and occurrence screening. These are rooted in the classical approaches of Deming (process improvement) and Crosby (zero defects).

Each approach has particular characteristic strengths and weaknesses. In order to make an effective contribution to patient care, it is essential that the characteristics of whichever method are understood. The appropriate use of whichever technique is employed is more important than choice of a particular technique.

As has been stated, one of the hardest tasks in quality improvement is to actually implement changes in practice. Within patient care, motivation to improve practice is generally high. However, as Deming noted, enthusiasm without appropriate tools and techniques is likely to lead quickly to disenchantment.

A further complication is that quality improvement is perceived by practitioners as a management activity. The biggest challenge is to provide clinicians with appropriate tools and techniques to make effective improvements to patient care without reducing their motivation by labelling quality assurance as a management activity divorced from patient care.

Bibliography

This bibliography provides a comprehensive list of all sources used in the preparation of this book, and the research on which it was based. It includes a collation of all the references from the individual chapters. Sources are arranged in alphabetical order of authors.

Abramson, J. H. (1984) *Survey Methods in Community Medicine*. Edinburgh: Churchill Livingstone.

Anderson, C. A., Cassidy, B. & Rivenburgh, P. (1991) Implementing continuous quality improvement (CQI) in hospitals: lessons learned from the International Quality Study. *Quality Assurance in Health Care*, **3**(3), 141–6.

Anglia and Oxford RHA & NHS Executive (1994) *Anglia & Oxford Clinical Audit in the Hospital and Community Health Services: Annual Report 1993/94*. Oxford: AORHA/NHSE.

Anglia and Oxford RHA & NHS Executive (1995) *The Role of Research and Audit in Evidence-Based Healthcare: Distinct but Linked*. Conference Proceedings, spring 1995.

Armstrong, R. & Morley, G. (1989) Working for patients: cost, control or both? *Health Services Management*, **85**, 5, 221–3.

Ashley, J. (1994) Linking ICD-9 to ICD-10: equivalence tables and the ICD-10 metadata file. *British Journal of Health Care Computing & Information Management*, **111**(10), 27–8.

Aukett, J. W. (1994) The development of clinical audit: use of a 'quality web' constructed for a community dental service. *International Journal of Health Care Quality Assurance*, **7**(1), 32–6.

Backer, T. E. (1995) Integrating behavioral and systems strategies to change clinical practice. *Journal of Quality Improvement*, **21**(7), 351–3.

Baker, A. (1976) The hospital advisory service. In: McLaughlin, G. (ed.), *A Question of Quality*. London: Oxford University Press, 203–16.

Baker, R. (1990) Problem solving with audit in general practice. *British Medical Journal*, **300**, 10 February.

Baker, R. & Fraser, R. (1993) MAAGs: The Eli Lilly National Clinical Audit Center. *International Journal of Health Care Quality Assurance*, **6**(3), 4–8.

Baker, R. & Presley, P. (1990) *The Practice Audit Plan*. Bristol: Severn Faculty of the Royal College of General Practitioners.

Baldeh, Y. (1995) Ethical considerations in the transfer of expert systems to developing countries. Prize-winning essay presented at ETHI-COMP '95, Leicester, March.

Banyard, R. F. (1989) Efficiency in the NHS: the search for a new paradigm. *Health Services Management*, **85**(2), 64–7.

Barrett, M. et al (1995) IT and IS in general practice. *Proceedings of the First International Symposium on Health Information Management Research, Sheffield, 5–7 April*, 112–118.

Batstone, G. F. (1990) Educational aspects of medical audit. *British Medical Journal*, **301**, 326–8.

Baugh, P. J., Fitzsimmons, D. A. & Walters, D. M. (1995) An examination of the introduction of case mix management systems in UK hospitals. *Proceedings of the First International Symposium on Health Information Management Research, University of Sheffield, 5–7 April*, 126–32.

Baugh, P. J., Gillies, A. C. & Jastrzebski, P. (1993) Combining knowledge-based and database technology in a tool for business planning. *Information and Software Technology*, **35**(3), 131–7.

Baugh, P. J. & Walters, D. M. (1994) The introduction of hospital information systems: the necessity for accomodation. Presented at the International System Dynamics Conference, University of Stirling.

Bell, L., Morris, B. & Brown, R. B. (1993) Devising a multidisciplinary audit tool. *International Journal of Health Care Quality Assurance*, **6**(4), 16–21.

Bennett, J. & Walshe, K. (1990) Occurrence screening as a method of audit. *British Medical Journal*, **300**, 1248–52.

Benson, T. & Neame, R. (1994) *Healthcare Computing*. Harlow: Longman.

Bernstein, S. J. & Hilborne, L. H. (1993) Clinical indicators: the road to quality of care? *Journal of Quality Improvement*, **19**(11), 501–9.

Besley, J. (1994) Interface audit and the shift of care. *Managing Audit in General Practice*, **11**(10), 6.

Bissell, A. F. (1990) Multipositional process evaluation: an example and some general guidelines. *Total Quality Management*, **1**(1), 95–100.

Black, N. A. & Moore, L. (1994) Comparative audit between hospitals: the example of appendectomy. *International Journal of Health Care Quality Assurance*, **7**(3), 11–15.

Blair-Fish, D. (1989) Medical audit: outcome measures needed. *British Medical Journal*, **299**, 2 December.

Blee, A. C. (1991) Health care in Finland. *Health Services Management*, **87**(1), 14–17.

Bowden, D. & Gumpert, R. (1988) Quality versus quantity in medicine. *RSA Journal*, April.

Bowden, D. & Walshe, K. (1991) When medical audit starts to count. *British Medical Journal*, **303**, 13 July.

Bowden, D., Williams, G. & Stevens, G. (1986) Medical quality assurance in Brighton: can American translate into English? In: Moores, B. (ed.), *Are They Being Served?* Oxford: Philip Allan, 104–14.

Boyce, J. (1990) The Audit Commission and the NHS. *Health Services Management*, **86**(4), 192–3.

Brennan, T. A., Localio, R. J. & Laird, N. L. (1989) Reliability and validity of judgements concerning adverse events suffered by hospitalised patients. *Medical Care*, **27**, 1148–58.

Brennan, T. A., Localio, R. J. & Leape, L. L. (1990) Identification of adverse events occurring during hospitalisation. *Annals of Internal Medicine*, **112**, 221–6.

Brook, R. H. (1991) Quality of care: do we care? *Annal of Medicine*, **115**(6), 486–90.

Brooks, T. (1992) Success through organisational audit. *Health Services Management*, **88**(8), November/December.

Brooks, T. (1992) Total quality management in the NHS. *Health Services Management*, **88**(2), April.

Brooks, T. (1994) *Quality Assurance and Improvement 1993–94* (NHS Handbook, 8th edn, ISBN 0 9520744 0 0).

Buck, N., Devlin, H. B. & Lunn, J. N. (1987) *Report of a Confidential Enquiry into Perioperative Deaths*. London: Nuffield Provincial Hospital Trust.

Bull, A. (1990) Doctors, management and audit. *Health Services Management*, **86**(6), December.

Burmeister, R. W. (1986) Occurrence screening: only the means to an end. *Quality, Risk and Cost Advisor*, **2**, 5–6.

Burns, L. R. & Beach, L. R. (1994) The quality improvement strategy. *Health Care Management Review*, **19**(2), 21–31.

California Medical Association and California Hospital Association (1977) *Report on the Medical Insurance Feasibility Study*. San Francisco: Sutter Publications.

Carlow, D. (1988) Occurrence screening can improve QA programs. *Dimensions Health Service*, **65**, 20–2.

Carroll, L., Thirlwall, M. & Wilson, A. (1994) Medical audit and the role of the facilitator. *International Journal of Health Care Quality Assurance,* **7**(3), 8–10.

Charlson, M. E., Pompei, P., Ales, K. L. & Mackenzie, C. R. (1987) A new method of classifying prognostic comorbidity in longitudinal studies: development and validation. *Journal of Chronic Disease,* **40**(5), 373–83.

Chassin, M. R. (1993) Improving quality of care with practice guidelines. *Frontiers of Health Services Managment,* **10**(1), 40–44.

Chisholm, S. & Gillies, A. C. (1994) A snapshot of the computerisation of general practice and the implications for training. *Auditorium,* **3**(1), 21–26.

Clarke, C. & Whitehead, A. G. W. (1981) The contribution of the Medical Services Group of the Royal College of Physicians to improvement in care. In: McLaughlin, G. (ed.), *Reviewing Practice in Medical Care: Steps to Quality Assurance.* London: Nuffield Provincial Hospital Trust.

Cleary, P. D. & McNeil, B. J. (1988) Patient satisfaction as an indicator of quality care. *Inquiry,* **25**, spring, 25–36.

Cohen, I, B. (1984) Florence Nightingale. *Scientific American,* (250), 98–107.

Coles, C. (1989) Self-assessment and medical audit: an educational approach. *British Medical Journal,* **299**, 807–88.

Collings, J. S. (1950) General practice in England today: a reconnaissance. *Lancet,* 558–85.

Conrad, D. A. (1993) The commentaries: a summary. *Frontiers of Health Services Management,* **10** (1), 39.

Craddick, J. W. (1979) The medical management analysis system: a professional liability warning mechanism. *Quality Review Bulletin,* April 1979.

Craddick, J. W. & Bader, B. (1983) *Medical Management Analysis: A Systematic Approach to Quality Assurance and Risk Management.* Auburn, CA: Joyce W. Craddick.

CRAG (1990) Confidentiality and medical audit: interim guidelines. *British Medical Journal,* **301**, 20 October.

CRAG (1990) *Report of a Working Group on Medical Audit and Information Technology,* JLC00224/090.

CRAG (1991) *Report of a Working Group on Access to Named Data by Management and Administration,* JLC00928/021.

CRAG (1993) *The Interface Between Clinical Audit and Management.*

CRAG (1993) *Consensus Statement—Depressive Illness: A Critical Review of Current Practice and the Way Ahead.*

CRAG (1995) *Clinical Guideline—Optimal Use of Donor Blood.*

CRAG (1995) *Clinical Guideline—Pressure Area Care.*

Crombie, I. K. & Davies, H. T. O. (1991) Audit in outpatients: entering the loop. *British Medical Journal,* **302**, 1437–9.

Crombie, I. K. & Davies, H. T. O. (1991) Computers in audit: servants or sirens? *British Medical Journal*, **303**, 403–4.

Crombie, I. K. & Davies, H. T. O. (1994) What shall we do with it? *Managing Audit in General Practice*, **11**(10), 8–10.

Crombie, I. K., Davies, H. T. O., Abraham, S. C. S. & du V. Florey, C. (1993) *The Audit Handbook: Improving Healthcare Through Clinical Audit.* Chichester: Wiley.

Crosby, P. B. (1986) *Quality is Free.* Maidenhead: McGraw-Hill.

Curl, M. & Robinson, D. (1994) Hand-held computers in clinical audit: a comparison with established paper and pencil methods. *International Journal of Health Care Quality Assurance*, **7**(3), 16–20.

Davies, A. R., Thomas Doyle, M. A., Lansky, D., Rutt, W., Orsoltis Stevic, M. & Doyle, J. B. (1994) Outcome assessment in clinical settings: a consensus statement on principles and best practices in project management. *Journal of Quality Improvement*, **20**(1), 6–16.

Davis, C. J., Gillies, A. C., Smith, P. & Thompson, J. B. (1993) Current practice in software quality and the impact of certification schemes. *Software Quality Journal*, **2**, 145–61.

Davison, A. J. (1990) Action in audit. *International Journal of Health Care Quality Assurance*, **3**(6), 14–16.

Dean J. A., Dean, A. G., Coulombie, D., Smith, D. C., Brendel, K. A. & Arner, T. G. (1995) *Epi Info Version 6: A Word-Processing, Database and Statistics Program for Epidemiology on Microcomputers.* Atlanta, GE: Centers for Disease Control and Prevention (available from USD Inc., 2075A West Park Place, Stone Mountain, GA 30087, USA; fax +404-469-0681).

Deming, W. E. (1986) *Out of the Crisis.* Cambridge, MA: MIT Center for Advanced Engineering.

Department of Health (1989) *Implications for Family Practitioner Committees* (NHS Review Working Paper 8). London: HMSO.

Department of Health (1989) *Medical Audit* (NHS Review Working Paper 6). London: HMSO.

Department of Health (1990) *Working for Patients—Framework for Information Systems: Overview.* London: HMSO.

Department of Health (1990) *Working for Patients—Framework for Information Systems: The Next Steps.* London: HMSO.

Department of Health (1990) *Working for Patients—Medical Audit: Guidance for Hospital Clinicians on the Use of Computers.* London: HMSO.

Department of Health (1992) *The Quality of Medical Care: Report of the Standing Medical Advisory Committee.* London: HMSO.

Department of Health (1994) *The Evolution of Clinical Audit.* London: NHS Management Executive/HMSO.

Difford, F. (1990) Defining essential data for audit in general practice. *British Medical Journal*, **300**, 92–4.

Dixon, N. (1991) *A Medical Audit Primer*. Hampshire: Healthcare Quality Quest.

Dollery, C. T. (1971) The quality of healthcare. In: McLaughlin, G. (ed.), *Challenges for Change*. London: Oxford University Press.

Donabedian, A. (1980) *The Definition of Quality and Approaches to Its Assessment*. Ann Arbor: Health Administration Press.

Eddy, D. M. (1990) Anatomy of a decision. *Journal of the American Medical Association*, **263**(3), 441–3.

Eddy, D. M. & Billings, J. (1988) The quality of medical evidence: implications for quality of care. *Health Affairs*, spring.

Ellis, B. W. (1988) Clinical audit. *British Journal of Hospital Medicine*, **39**, 187.

Ellis, B. W. (1989) How to set up an audit. *British Medical Journal*, **298**, 1635–7.

Ellis, B. W., Michie, H. R., Esulfali, S. T., Pyper, R. J. D. & Dudley, H. A. F. (1987) Development of a microcomputer-based system for surgical audit and patient administration: a review. *Journal of the Royal Society of Medicine*, **80**, March.

Ellis, N. T. (1995) Audit of audit: a survey of audit practice in the four counties, Anglia and Oxford region. *Auditorium*, **4**(2), 8–10.

Ellis, N. T. & Gillies, A. C. (1995) The reality of medical audit: the Oxford experience. *Proceedings of the First International Symposium on Health Information Management, Sheffield, 5–7 April*, 34–43.

Epstein, A. M. (1990) The outcomes movement: will it get us where we want to go? *New England Journal of Medicine*, **323**, 266–9.

Farquhar, W. J. (1992) Audit in Scotland. *Medical Audit News*, **2**(2), 45–7.

Fernandez, C. (1991) Medical audit in the acute services. *International Journal of Health Care Quality Assurance*, **4**(4), 12–14.

Firth-Cozens, J. & Storer, D. (1992) Registrars' and senior registrars' perceptions of their audit activities. *Quality in Health Care*, **1**, 161–4.

Fisher, R. B. & Dearden, C. H. (1990) Improving the care of patients with major trauma in the accident and emergency department. *British Medical Journal*, **300**, 1560–3.

Fitzsimmons, D. (1995) Next generation UK healthcare systems. In: *Business Research Yearbook. Vol. II: Global Business Perspectives*. Maryland: University Press of America Inc., 505–9.

Fitzsimmons, D., Baugh, P. J. & Walters, D. (1995) SSM: a guiding light in the introduction to hospital case-mix management systems. In: *Critical Issues in Systems Theory*. New York: Plenum, 603–8.

Fowkes, F. G. R. & McPake, B. I. (1986) Regional variations in outpatient activity in England and Wales. *Community Medicine*, **8**, 286–91.

Fox, D., Reynolds, B., Callaghan, C. & Strickland, T. (1992) Using occurrence screening in medical audit. *Network*, **5**, January.

Franco, L. M., Richardson, P., Reynolds, J. & Meeraj, K. (1993) *Management Advancement Program Vol. 5: Performance Indicators*. Geneva: Aga Khan Foundation/World Health Organization.

Gabbay, J., McNicol, M. C., Spiby, J., Davies, S. C. & Layton, A. J. (1990) What did audit achieve? Lessons from preliminary evaluation of a year's medical audit. *British Medical Journal*, **301**, 526–9.

Garvin, D. (1984) What does quality mean? *Sloan Management Review*, **4**, 125–31.

Gillies, A. C. (1990) The quality of images as a measurement of image processing operator performance in fringe analysis. *Journal of Photographic Science*, **38**, 135–9 (based on a paper presented at the Royal Photographic Society Symposium on the Quantification of Images, Cambridge, 1989).

Gillies, A. C. (1992) Modelling software quality in the commercial environment. *Software Quality Journal*, **1**, 175–91.

Gillies, A. C. (1994) Manufacturing expert systems. Presented at the World Congress on Expert Systems, Lisbon.

Gillies, A. C. (1994) Quality assurance in expert systems. Presented at the World Congress on Expert Systems, Lisbon.

Gillies, A. C. (1994) LOQUM: locally defined quality modelling. *Total Quality Management*, **5**(3), 71–75.

Gillies, A. C. (1994) METACASE: one step beyond? Invited presentation at First International Symposium on MetaCase, Sunderland.

Gillies, A. C. (1994) Computerization of general practice: most efficacious in every case? Presentation to the Preston Group of the British Computing Society.

Gillies, A. C. (1994) On the usability of software for medical audit. *Auditorium*, **3**(1), 14–20.

Gillies, A. C. (1995) The computerisation of general practice: an IT perspective. *Journal of Information Technology*, **10**(1), 75–85.

Gillies, A. C. (1995) *Information Management for Medical Audit: A Handbook*. Department of Postgraduate Medical Education and Training, John Radcliffe Hospital, Oxford.

Gillies, A. C. (1996) *Software Quality*, 2nd edn. London: Chapman & Hall.

Gillies, A. C. (1996) Improving patient care in the UK: clinical audit in the Oxford Region. *International Journal of Health Care Quality Assurance*, **8**(2), 141–52.

Gillies, A. C. & Baldeh, Y. (1995) Twenty years on from MYCIN: the lessons that should have been learnt in methods, co-operative decision-making and validation for medical applications. *Romanian Journal of Applied Medical Informatics*, **1**(1), 1–10.

Gillies, A. C. & Baugh, P. (1994) *Excel in Health Care*. London: Chapman & Hall.

Gillies, A. C., Smith, P. & Lansbury, M. (1994) Quality improvement in knowledge-based systems. Presented at the Fourth European Conference on Software Quality, Basle.

Glass, R. E. & Thomas, P. A. (1987) Surgical audit in a district general hospital: a stimulus for improving patient care. *Annals of the Royal College of Surgeons of England*, **69**, 135–9.

Godber, G. (1976) The confidential enquiry into maternal deaths. In: McLaughlin, G. A. (ed.), *A Question of Quality*. London: Oxford University Press, 24–33.

Goldberg, H. I. (1993) Should we be implementing untested guidelines? *Frontiers of Health Services Management*, **10**(1), 45–7.

Grubb, P. A., Dixon, R. M., Camplin, D. A. & Takang, A. A. (1995) Pulling the strands together: what the future has in store for medical informatics technology. *Proceedings of a Conference on Healthcare Computing*, Harrogate: 561–7.

Gumpert, R. & Lyons, C. (1990) Setting up a district audit programme. *British Medical Journal*, **301**, 162–6.

Hall, H. (1979) Say 'No' to audit. *World Medicine*, **14**, 21–2.

Hancock, B. D. (1990) Audit of major colorectal and biliary surgery to reduce rates of wound infection. *British Medical Journal*, **301**, 911–12.

Harman, D. & Martin, G. (1992) Managers and medical audit. *Health Services Management*, **88**(2), 27–9.

Harris, N., Hindhaugh, J. & Thomas, F. (1991) Quality in the NHS: real or illusionary change? *Health Services Management*, **87**(2), 81.

Heath, D. A. (1990) Random review of hospital patient records. *British Medical Journal*, **300**, 651–3.

Hepworth, J. B. & Urquhart, C. J. (1995) The value of databases in clinical decision making: audit tools to enhance the outcomes of information delivery. *Proceedings of a Conference on Healthcare Computing*, Harrogate, 45–52.

Higgins, A. F., Lewis, A., Noone, P. & Hole, M. L. (1980) Single and multiple dose cotrimoxazole and metronidazole in colorectal surgery. *British Medical Journal*, **67**, 90–2.

Honigsbaum, F. (1993) How the health service evolved. In: *NHS Handbook*, 8th edn. London: NHS.

Hopkins, A. (1991) Approaches to medical audit. *Journal of Epidemiology & Community Health*, **45**, 1–3.

Hopkins, A. (ed.) (1994) *Professional and Managerial Aspects of Clinical Audit*. London: Royal College of Physicians.

Hopkins, J. (1989) Methodologies. *Quality, Risk and Cost Advisor*, **5**, 7.

Hughes, J. & Humphrey, C. (1990) What is medical audit? In: *Medical*

Audit in General Practice: A Guide to the Literature (Medical Audit Series 3), August.

Hughes, J. & Humphrey, C. (1990) Themes and further questions. In: *Medical Audit in General Practice: A Guide to the Literature* (Medical Audit Series 3), August.

Hughes, J. & Humphrey, C. (1990) References. In: *Medical Audit in General Practice: A Guide to the Literature* (Medical Audit Series 3), August.

Hunt, V. & Legg, F. (1994) *Clinical Audit: A Basic Introduction.* Oxford University: Regional Postgraduate Medical Education & Training Office.

Iezzoni, L. I. (ed.) (1994) *Risk Adjustment for Measuring Health Care Outcomes.* Ann Arbor: Health Administration Press.

Irozuru, E., Baugh, P. J., Gillies, A. C. & Rae, J. (1995) Organizations as information networks: a strategy for IS management in a DHA. *Proceedings of the First International Symposium on Health Information Management Research, Sheffield, 5–7 April,* 56–66.

Ishikawa, K. (1985) *What is Total Quality Control?—The Japanese Way.* Englewood Cliffs, NJ: Prentice Hall.

International Standards Organisation (1986) *ISO 8042: Quality Vocabulary.* Geneva: ISO (available from BSI, London).

International Standards Organisation (1994) *ISO 9000 Series: Standards for Quality Management Systems.* Geneva: ISO (available from BSI, London).

Izzard, H. (1994) Hard centres. *Health Service Journal,* **104**, 53–95.

Jackson, P. (1993) Quality audit in gynaecology. *International Journal of Health Care Quality Assurance,* **6**(2), 9–11.

James, B. C. (1993) Implementing practice guidelines through clinical quality improvement. *Frontiers of Health Services Management,* **10**(1), 3–37.

Jonas, S. & Rosenberg, S. N. (1986) Measurement and control in the quality of health care. In: Jonas, S. (ed.), *Health Care Delivery in the United States.* New York: Springer Verlag, 416–64.

Jordan, H. S., Straus, J. H. & Bailit, M. H. (1995) Reporting and using health plan performance information in Massachusetts. *Journal of Quality Improvement,* **21**(4), 167–77.

Juran, J. M. (1979) *Quality Control Handbook,* 3rd edn. Maidenhead: McGraw-Hill.

Jutras, D. (1993) Guidelines workshop: clinical practice guidelines as legal norms. *Canadian Medical Association Journal,* **148**(6), 905–8.

Kahn, M. G., Steib, S. A., Spitznagel, E. L., Dunagen, W. C. & Fraser, V. J. (1995) Improvement in user performance following development and routine use of an expert system. Presented at the MedInfo '95 Conference.

Kane-Berman, J. (1995) Performance indicators: adding value to hospital management. Presented at the MedInfo '95 Conference.

Kanji, G. K. (1990) Total quality management: the second industrial revolution. *Total Quality Management*, **1**(1), 3–12.

Kaplan, B. (1965) Barriers to medical computing: history, diagnosis and therapy for the medical computing 'lag'. Presented at the Ninth Annual Symposium on Computer Applications in Medical Care.

Kelly, S. (1994) Who's afraid of the big bad computer? *Managing Audit in General Practice*, **111**(10), 11–12.

Kibbe, D. C., Kaluzny, A. D. & McLaughlin, C. P. (1994) Integrating guidelines with continuous quality improvement: doing the right thing the right way to achieve the right goals. *Journal on Quality Improvement*, **20**(4), 181–91.

King, J. G. (1993) The relevence of practical experience to American hospitals. *Frontiers of Health Services Management*, **10**(1), 48–50.

Kitchenham, B. (1989) Software quality assurance. *Microprocessors and Microcomputers*, **13**(6), 373–81.

Koska, M. T. (1989) Satisfaction data: patient perception is reality. *Hospitals*, **63**, 40.

Lal, S., Griffiths, A. & Rothwell, P. (1990) Outpatients and quality: the need for information. *Health Services Management*, **86**(5), 231–5.

Lamb, M. (1995) Patient outcome by discharge: an integrated multi-disciplinary audit. Presented at a Conference on Healthcare Computing, 1995, Harrogate, 53–61.

Lancet Editorial (1990) Legislated clinical medicine. *Lancet*, **335**, 1004–6.

Lane, R. L. & Lurie, N. (1992) Appropriate effectiveness: a tale of carts and horses. *Quality Review Bulletin*, **18**, 322–6.

Lear, P. (1989) Caring for the 1990s in the USSR. *Health Services Management*, **85**(4), 164–8.

Lembcke, P. A. (1967) Evolution of the medical audit. *Journal of the American Medical Association*, **199**, 111–18.

Lewis, M. (1990) Standards and nursing audit. *International Journal of Health Care Quality Assurance*, **3**(6), 21–32.

Lindgren, B. (1974) The Swedish healthcare system. *British Medical Journal*, **30**(3), 74–9.

Lohr, K. N. (1988) Outcome measurement: concepts and questions. *Inquiry*, **25**, 37–50.

Lohr, K. N. & Schroeder, S. A. (1990) A strategy for quality in Medicare. *New England Journal of Medicine*, **323**, 266–9.

Lomas, J., Enkin, M., Anderson, G. M. et al (1991) Opinion leaders versus audit and feedback to implement practice guidelines: delivery after previous cesarian section. *Journal of the American Medical Association*, **265**, 2202–7.

Lomas, J. & Haynes, R. B. (1988) A taxonomy and critical review of tested strategies for the application of clinical practice recommendations: from 'official' to 'individual' clinical policy. *American Journal of Preventive Medicine*, **4** (suppl.), 77–94.

Long, A. (1994) *IFMH Study Day: Outcome Measurement*. 15 November.

Lonsdale, M. (1993) Auditing for fundholding success. *Health Services Management*, **89**(8), 14–15.

Lord, J. & Littlejohs, P. (1994) Secret garden. *Health Service Journal*, **104**, 5417.

Lough, J. R. M. & McKay, J. (1992) CRAG Occasional Paper—Audit and training: a model for general practice. *Audit Symposium*, **24**.

Lyons, C. & Gumpert, R. (1990) Medical audit data: counting is not enough. *British Medical Journal*, **300**, 1563–6.

Matchet, A. & Rose, P. (1992) Medical audit in the quality process: a practical implementation. *International Journal of Health Care Quality Assurance*, **5**(6), 15–17.

McConnachiie, R. W. (1990) Organisation of audit in North Derbyshire Health Authority. *British Medical Journal*, **300**, 1566–8.

McKee, C. M., Lauglo, M. & Lessof, L. (1989) Medical audit: a review. *Journal of the Royal Society of Medicine*, **82**, 474–8.

McKee, C. M., Dixon, J. & Chenet, L. (1994) Making routine data adequate to support clinical audit: unambiguous definitions are needed. *British Medical Journal*, **309**, 1246–7.

McLaughlin, G. (1976) Introduction and perspectives. In: McLaughlin, G. (ed.), *A Question of Quality*. London: Oxford University Press, 3–20.

McNicol, G. P. (1979) A rather sad document. *British Medical Journal*, **2**, 844–8.

McPherson, K., Strong, P. M., Epstein, A. & Jones, L. (1981) Regional variations in the use of common surgical procedures: within and between England and Wales, Canada and the USA. *Society for Science in Medicine*, **15A**, 273–88.

Metcalfe, D. H. H. (1989) Audit in general practice. *British Medical Journal*, **299**, 25 November.

Michaels, J. (1989) Best documented practice. *British Medical Journal*, **299**, 15 July.

Miles, A. (1994), From rhetoric to reality. *Managing Audit in General Practice*, **111**(10), 19–22.

Mitchell, M. W. & Fowkes, F. G. R. (1985) Audit reviewed: does feedback on performance change clinical behaviour? *Journal of the Royal College of Physicians of London*, **19**(4), 251–4.

Mooney, G. & Ryan, M. (1991) Rethinking medical audit: the goal is efficiency. Department of Public Health and Economics, University of Aberdeen.

Mosley, J. & Fairbanks, R. (1992) Using audit in a district-wide management system. *Health Services Management*, **88**(5), 27–9.

Moss, F. & Smith, R. (1991) From audit to quality and beyond. *British Medical Journal*, **303**, 199–200.

Mourin, K. (1975) Audit in general practice. *Journal of the Royal College of General Practitioners*, **25**, 682–3.

Mugford, M., Banfield, P. & O'Hanlon, M. (1991) Effects of feedback of information on clinical practice: a review. *British Medical Journal*, **303**, 398–402.

National Consumer Council (1992) *Quality Standards in the NHS: The Consumer Focus*. PD18/92/HIa, September.

Neave, H. R. (1987) Deming's 14 points for management. *The Statistician*, **36**, 561–70.

NHS IMG (1994) *Clinical Workstations: Focus for the Future.*

NHS Management Executive (1993) *Meeting and Improving Standards in Healthcare: a Policy Statement on the Development of Clinical Audit.* EL993/59, July.

NHS Management Executive (1994) Clinical audit: 1994/95 and beyond. *Executive Letter*, 94, 20.

NHS Management Executive & Anglia and Oxford Regional Health Authority (1994) *Clinical Audit in the Hospital and Community Health Services—Annual Report 1993/94; Forward Programme 1994/95*. July.

NHS Management Executive & IMG (1994) *This is the IMG 1994: A Guide to the IMG of the NHS Management Executive*. October.

NHS Management Executive & IMG (1994) *Introduction to Data Protection in the NHS.*

NHS Management Executive & IMG (1995) *So you want your computers to talk to each other? A Manager's Guide to Applying NHS IT Standards in Procurements. STEP = Standards Enforcement in Procurement.* March.

NHS Management Executive & IMG (1995) *NHS IT Standards in Procurement—Version 2.0*. E5184, March.

Nichol, D. K. (1989) Working for patients: the role of managers in implementing the White Paper. *Health Services Management*, **85**(3), 107–9.

Nixon, S. J. (1990) Defining essential hospital data. *British Medical Journal*, **300**, 380–2.

Norman, L. A., Hardin, P. A., Lester, E., Stinton, S. & Vincent, E. C. (1995) Computer-assisted quality improvement in an ambulatory care setting: a follow-up report. *The Joint Commission Journal*, **21**(3), 116–131.

Oakland, J. (1989) *Total Quality Management*. London: Heinemann.

Office of Health Economics (1989) *Compendium of Health Statistics*. London: HMSO.

O'Leary, D. S. (1987) The Joint Commission looks to the future. *Journal of the American Medical Association*, **258**, 951–2.

O'Leary, D. S. (1993) The measurement mandate: report card day is coming. *Journal of Quality Improvement*, **19**(11), 487–91.

Omachonu, V. K. (1990) Quality of care and the patient: new criteria for evaluation. *Health Care Management Review*, **15**(4), 43–50.

Ovretveit, J. (1990) What is quality in health services? *Health Services Management*, **86**(3), 132–3.

Oxford Regional Health Authority (1993) *Medical Audit in the Hospital and Community Health Services—Annual Report 1992/93; Forward Programme 1993/94.*

Palmer, R. H. (1996) Measuring clinical performance to provide information for quality improvement. *Quality Management in Health Care*, **4**(2), 1–6.

Panniers, T. L. & Newlander, J. (1986) The adverse patient occurrences inventory: validity, reliability and implications. *Quality Review Bulletin*, **12**, 311–15.

Parry, K. M. (1989) Medical education report—the curriculum for the year 2000. *Proceedings of a Conference of the Association for the Study of Medical Education, September 1988*, **23**, 301–4.

Perry, S. & Wilkinson, S. L. (1992) The technology assessment and practice guidelines forum: a modified group judgement method. *International Journal of Technology Assessment in Healthcare*, **18**(2), 289–300.

Peterken, L. E. (1990) General management in Glasgow: the search for efficiency. *Health Services Management*, **86**(5), 216–20.

Pollock, A. V. (1989) The rise and fall of the random trial in surgery. *Theory in Surgery*, **4**, 163–70.

Puntis, J. W. L., Holden, C. E., Smallman, S., Kinkel, Y., George, R. H. & Booth, I. W. (1990) Staff training: a key factor in reducing intravascular catheter sepsis. *Archives of Diseases in Children*, **65**, 335–7.

Read, J. D. (1990) The READ clinical classification (READ codes). *Proceedings of the Medical Informatics Europe Conference*, 645–649.

Reerink, E. (1990) Improving the quality of hospital services in the Netherlands. *Quality Assurance in Health Care*, **2**(1), 13–19.

Reerink, E. (1991) Arcadia revisited: quality assurance in hospitals in the Netherlands. *British Medical Journal*, **302**, 15 June.

Reinertsen, J. L. (1993) Outcomes management and continuous quality improvement: the compass and the rudder. *Quality Review Bulletin*, **19**, 5–7.

Renwick, P. A. (1992) Quality assurance in health care: the theoretical context. *International Journal of Health Care Quality Assurance*, **5**(5), 29–34.

Rigby, M., McBride, A. & Shiels, C. (1992) *Computers in Medical Audit.* London: University of Keele/West Midlands RHA/Royal Society of Medicine Services Ltd.

Roberts, C. J. (1988) Annotation: towards the more effective use of diagnostic radiology, a review of the Royal College of Radiologists—working party on the more effective use of diagnostic radiology, 1976–88. *Clinical Radiology,* **39**, 3–6.

Roberts, J. S., Coale, J. G. & Redman, R. R. (1987) A history of the Joint Commission of the Accreditation of Hospitals. *Journal of the American Medical Association,* **258**, 936–40.

Robinson, M. L. (1988) Sneak preview: JCAHO's quality indicators. *Hospitals,* **62**, 38–43.

Rohrer, J. E. (1989) The secret of medical management. *Health Care Management Review,* **14**(3), 7–13.

Royal College of Physicians of London (1989) *Medical Audit—A First Report: What, Why and How?* London: RCPL.

Royal College of Physicians of London (1993) *Medical Audit—A Second Report.* London: RCPL.

Royal College of Psychiatrists (1989) *Preliminary Report on Auditing.* London: RCS.

Royal College of Radiologists (1979) National study of preoperative chest radiology. *Lancet,* **ii**, 83–6.

Royal College of Surgeons of England (1989) *Guidelines to Clinical Audit in Surgical Practice.* London: RCSE.

Royal College of Surgeons of England (1991) *Guidelines for Surgical Audit by Computer.* London: RCSE.

Ruscon, M. N. J. (1990) Audit in general practice. *British Medical Journal,* **300**, 6 January.

Sale, D. (1990) Quality now and in the future. In: *Essentials of Nursing Management—Quality Assurance.* London: Macmillan.

Sale, D. (1990) Quality Patient Care Scale (Qualpacs). In: *Essentials of Nursing Management—Quality Assurance.* London: Macmillan.

Sanderson, H. (1987) Potential benefits for patient care from computing. *Community Medicine,* **9**(3), 236–46.

Schroeder, S. A. (1987) Outcome assessment 70 years later: are we ready? *New England Journal of Medicine,* **316**, 160–1.

Schult, T. & Janetzko, D. (1993) Moving towards expert systems globally in the 21st century—Case-based expert system shells: first and second generation. Presented at an Expert Systems Conference, Lisbon.

Schumacher, D. N., Parker, B. & Kofie, V. (1987) Severity of illness index and the adverse patient occurrence index: a reliability study and policy implications. *Medical Care,* **25**, 695–704.

Sechrest, L., Backer, T. E., Rogers, E. M., Campbell, T. R. & Grady, M. L. (eds) (1994) *Effective Dissemination of Clinical and Health Information.* Rockville, MD: US Department of Health and Human Services.

Seddon, T. D. S. (1989) Improving our health service. In from the cold: the essential twins, quality assurance and information systems. *New Zealand Medical Journal,* **102,** 644–47.

Semple, E. E., Gregson, K. E. & McEwen, J. (1993) CRAG Occasional Paper—A clinical audit support group: moving with the times. *Audit Symposium,* **38.**

Semple, E. E., Gregson, K. E. & McEwen, J. (1994) The changing role of an audit support group. *Scottish Medical Journal,* **39**(1), 21–3.

Shapleigh, C. (1991) Patient data critical to hospital-wide quality. *Healthcare Financial Management,* **45,** June, 80–8.

Sharp, T. & Kilvington, J. (1993) Towards integrative audit: a partnership for quality. *International Journal of Health Care Quality Assurance,* **6**(4), 12–15.

Sharples, P. M., Storey, A., Aynsley-Green, A. & Eyre, J. A. (1990) Avoidable factors contributing to death of children with head injury. *British Medical Journal,* **300,** 87–91.

Shaw, C. D. (1980) Aspects of audit. 5: Looking forward to audit. *British Medical Journal,* **280,** 1509–11.

Shaw, C. D. (1988) Clinical outcome indicators. *Health Trends,* **21,** 37–40.

Shaw, C. D. (1989) *Medical Audit: A Hospital Handbook.* London: King's Fund Centre.

Shaw, C. D. (1990) Criterion-based audit. *British Medical Journal,* **300,** 649–51.

Shaw, C. D. (1991) Specifications for hospital medical audit. *Health Services Management,* **87**(3), 124–5.

Shaw, C. D. & Costain, D. W. (1989) Guidelines for medical audit: seven principles. *British Medical Journal,* **299,** 19 August.

Slee, V. N. (1967) In: Eisele, C. W. (ed.), *The Medical Staff and the Modern Hospital.* New York: McGraw-Hill.

Smith, C. W. (1950) *Florence Nightingale.* London: Constable.

Smith, P. (1992) Collecting clinical information for audit: solving the problem. *International Journal of Health Informatics,* **2**(2), 9–13.

Smith, T. (1990) Audit: quality costs more, not less. *British Medical Journal,* **300,** 24 February.

Smith, T. (1990) Medical audit: closing the feedback loop is vital. *British Medical Journal,* **300,** 65.

Smitts, H. L. (1981) The PRSO in perspective. *New England Journal of Medicine,* **305,** 253–9.

Sonnenberg, F. A., Hagerty, C. G. & Kulikowski, C. A. (1994) An architecture for knowledge-based construction of decision models. *Medical Decision Making*, **14**(1), 27–39.

South East Thames Regional Health Authority (1989) *Briefing: New Medical Audit Process for Britain*. Bexhill: SET RHA.

Spencer-Jones, N. (1993) IT for care, efficiency and cultural change. *Health Services Management*, **89**(7), 22–3.

Spicer, J., Walker, S. & Telford, B. (1992) Quality assurance ward audit. *International Journal of Health Care Quality Assurance*, **5**(1), 27–92.

Standing Committee on Postgraduate Medical Education (1989) *Medical Audit: The Educational Implications*. London: SCOPME.

Stevens, G. & Bennett, J. (1989) Clinical audit: occurrence screening for quality assurance. *Health Services Management*, **85**(4), 178–81.

Stevens, G., Wickings, I. & Bennett, J. (1988) Medical quality assurance: research in Brighton Health Authority. *International Journal of Health Care Quality Assurance*, **1**, 5–11.

Stevens, J. B. (1989) Some lessons from France. *Health Services Management*, **85**(5), 224–7.

Stewart Orr, J. (1989) Integrated system philosophy for integrated hospitals. *Health Services Management*, **85**(5), 219–20.

Stock, S., Young, M., Hardiman, P. J. & Petty, A. H. (1985) A microcomputer based system for surgical audit. *British Journal of Clinical Practice*, July, 261–6.

Strauss, M. B. (1968) *Familiar Medical Quotations*. Boston: Little, Brown.

Tan, J. H. T. & Hanna, J. (1994) Integrating health care with information technology: knitting patient information through networking. *Health Care Management Review*, **19**(2), 72–80.

Thomas, P. (1988) Decision making and the management of change in the NHS. *Health Services Management*, **88**(4), 28–31.

Thomasson, G. O. (1994) Participatory risk management: promoting physician compliance with practice guidelines. *Journal on Quality Improvement*, **20**(6), 317–29.

Todd, J. S. (1993) Quest for quality of cost containment. *Frontiers of Health Services Management*, **10**(1), 51–3.

Tyndall, R., Kennedy, S., Naylor, S. & Pajack, F. (1990) *Computers in Medical Audit*. London: Royal Society of Medicine.

Van Cleave, E. F. (1989) Uses of risk adjusted outcomes in quality assurance monitoring. In: Spath, P. L. (ed.), *Innovations in Healthcare Quality Management*. Chicago: American Hospital Publishing Inc., 1–9.

Walczak, R. (1984) Occurrence screening: is it worth it? *Quality, Risk and Cost Advisor*, **1**, 1–7.

Walshe, K. (1993) *Making Audit Work: Guidelines on Selecting, Planning, Implementing and Evaluating Audit Projects*. CASPE Research.

Weale, F. E. (1988) Why on earth do surgeons need quality assurance? *Annals of the Royal College of Surgeons of England*, **70**, 261.

Webb, S. J., Dowell, A. C. & Heywood, P. (1991) Survey of general practice audit in Leeds. *British Medical Journal*, **302**, 390–3.

Wennberg, J. E., Freeman, J. L. & Culp, W. J. (1987) Are hospital services rationed in New Haven or over-utilised in Boston? *Lancet*, 1185–8.

White, D. (1994) Audit: an answer to all your needs. *Managing Audit in General Practice*, **11**(10), 4–4.

Whitehead, T. (1976) Surveying the performance of pathological laboritories. In: McLaughlin, G. (ed.), *A Question of Quality*. London: Oxford University Press, 97–117.

Whitehouse, J. M. A. (1989) Best documented practice. *British Medical Journal*, **298**, 10 June.

Whitford, D. L. & Southern, A. J. (1994) Audit of secondary prophylaxis after myocardial infarction. *British Medical Journal*, **309**, 1268–9.

Wilkin, D. & Smith, A. G. (1987) Variation in general practitioners referral rates to consultants. *Journal of the Royal College of General Practitioners*, **37**, 350–3.

Williams, J. G., Kingham, M. J., Morgan, J. M. & Davies, A. B. (1990) Retrospective review of hospital patient records. *British Medical Journal*, **300**, 991–3.

Williamson, J. D. (1973) Quality control, medical audit and the general practitioner. *Journal of the Royal College of General Practitioners*, **23**, 697–706.

Williamson, J. D. (1991) Providing quality care. *Health Services Management*, **87**(1), 18–23.

Wilson, N. & McClean, S. (1994) *Questionnaire Design: A Practical Introduction*. University of Ulster.

Winsten, J. A. (1976) Regulating shared health facilities in New York City. In: Greene, R. (ed.), *Assuring Quality in Medical Care*. Cambridge, MA: Ballinger, 195–211.

World Health Organization (1994) *Health for All Database*, World Wide Web. Geneva: WHO.

Young, D. W. (1991) Can we get doctors to use computers? *Health Services Management*, **87**(3), 116–18.

Index

Index compiled by Liz Granger